Chair Tai Chi for Seniors Over 60

An Illustrated 4-Week Guide of Easy, Safe 10-Minute Daily Seated
Exercises to Improve Mobility, Build Balance and Boost Mental Clarity

Xian Ming

Disclaimer

This book is intended for general informational and educational purposes only. The exercises and guidance contained in this publication are not a substitute for professional medical advice, diagnosis, or treatment. Always consult your physician or qualified healthcare provider before beginning any new exercise program, particularly if you have a pre-existing medical condition, recent injury, or surgery.

The author and publisher assume no responsibility for any injury, loss, or damage incurred as a result of the use or application of information contained in this book.

Dedication

For every person who has ever been told, by circumstance, by pain, or by the quiet voice of doubt, that their body is no longer capable of something beautiful.

It is.

This book is for the student who showed up on a Tuesday morning not knowing why, and found something worth returning to. For the hands that shook on the first day and steadied by the fourth week. For the bodies that have carried decades of living and still, every single morning, choose to keep moving.

And for those who loved someone enough to place this book in their hands.

May every page remind you that gentleness is not weakness, that slowness is not failure, and that ten quiet minutes given to yourself each day is one of the most courageous things a person can do.

This is for you.

Table of Contents

Introduction: Ten Minutes That Can Change Everything

This book began the way most useful things begin: in a room full of people who needed something that did not yet exist in quite the right form.

The room was a community center. The people were eleven seniors, ranging in age from 64 to 81, who had signed up for a gentle movement class with varying degrees of enthusiasm and skepticism. Some had been sent by their doctors. Some had come because a friend was coming. One had arrived simply because she needed somewhere to be on Tuesday mornings.

What they had in common was this: they were living in bodies that had changed on them. Joints that used to move freely now protested. Balance that used to be automatic had become something they actively thought about, sometimes anxiously, every time they moved through a space. Several had stopped doing things they once loved, not because they had decided to stop, but because the body had gradually, quietly made those things feel too uncertain or too painful to continue.

What they needed was not a workout. They needed a practice that met them exactly where they were, respected what their bodies could do today, and offered genuine benefit without requiring them to become something they were not.

Chair Tai Chi was that practice. It still is.

What This Book Offers

You're holding a practical, four-week roadmap designed specifically for bodies that have lived a little. We aren't training for the Olympics here. We're training for life; for better balance when you reach for a cup, for less stiffness when you wake up, and for the quiet confidence of knowing you can move freely again.

No prior experience is required. No flexibility, strength, or fitness level is a prerequisite. All you need is a sturdy chair, a small amount of clear floor space, and the willingness to show up for ten minutes a day and pay attention.

Who This Book Is For

This book is for you if you are over 60 and looking for a movement practice that is safe, accessible, and genuinely effective. It is for you if you live with limited mobility, chronic pain, balance concerns, arthritis, cardiovascular issues, or the early signs of cognitive change. It is equally for you if you are in good health and simply want a daily practice that keeps you that way.

It is for you if you have tried exercise programs before and stopped. It is for you if you have never exercised regularly. It is for you if you are returning to movement after illness, injury, or loss.

Chair Tai Chi does not care about your history. It only cares about where you are right now, and where you would like to go from here.

How to Use This Book

Read Chapters 1 and 2 before attempting any practice. They contain the foundational understanding and practical preparation that make every session safer and more effective. Chapter 3 introduces the core principles of breath, posture, and basic movement. Spend at least two to three days with it before beginning the four-week program in Chapter 5.

Chapters 5 through 8 are your weekly practice guides. Use them day by day, reading each movement fully before attempting it. Chapter 9 is a reference for specific health needs. Return to it as a supplement to your weekly practice whenever relevant. Chapter 10 is for after the four-week program ends and is best read during Week 4 as you begin thinking about what comes next.

One last tip: I know how frustrating it is to break your concentration just to flip pages and remember what comes next. That's why I added **The 10-Minute Daily Quick Reference Guide** in the Bonus section of this book. Once you read through a weekly chapter, just lay those summary pages flat next to your chair. You'll be able to see your entire daily routine at a single glance.

How to Pace Yourself Over the Next Four Weeks

In my 15 years of teaching older adults, I've seen a lot of people start a new routine with great enthusiasm, only to quit a week later because they pushed too hard. We are going to do things differently.

Before you turn to Week 1, here is exactly how you should approach your practice:

- **Practice 5 days a week, not 7.** Your body actually builds strength and improves its balance during the time you rest. Take two days off every week. You can take the weekends off, or simply rest whenever your body asks for a break.

- **Keep it to 10 minutes.** Don't try to speed through the movements just to check them off a list. Moving slowly is the whole point. If it takes you 12 minutes because you are taking deep breaths and taking your time, that is perfectly fine.

- **Find your best time of day.** I usually tell my students to practice mid-morning, right around 9:00 or 10:00 AM. By then, the initial stiffness of waking up has worn off, but the afternoon fatigue hasn't hit yet. However, if you prefer evenings, practice 1 hour before bed to wind down.

- **Treat the repetitions as suggestions.** If I tell you to do 5 arm swings, but your shoulder says 3 is enough today, then 3 is your perfect number. Never argue with your joints.

Before You Begin

Find your chair. Place it in a quiet space with a few feet of clear floor around it. Sit down. Feel your feet on the floor.

Take one slow breath in through your nose and release it completely through your mouth.

You have already begun.

Chapter 1: The Power of Chair Tai Chi

There is a moment that happens in almost every Chair Tai Chi class I have ever taught. It usually occurs somewhere around the third or fourth session. A student who came in hunched, hesitant, and a little skeptical will suddenly sit up straighter during a breathing exercise. Their shoulders drop. Their jaw unclenches. Their eyes get a little softer. They are not thinking about their aching knees or the doctor's appointment next Tuesday. For those ten minutes, they are simply here, breathing, moving, alive in their body in a way that feels both new and strangely familiar.

That moment is the power of Chair Tai Chi.

It is not a dramatic power. It does not announce itself with fireworks or the burn of a hard workout. It arrives quietly, the way good things often do for people who have lived long enough to appreciate quiet. And once it arrives, it tends to stay.

This book is built around that moment and around helping you find it for yourself. It doesn't matter if you're 62 or 85. It doesn't matter if you used to run marathons or if you've never done a push-up in your life. This practice meets you where you are. All it asks is ten minutes a day and a willingness to show up.

The four-week program in these pages is designed to meet you exactly where you are. Not where you were ten years ago. Not where you think you should be. Right here, right now, in the body you have today. That is where we begin.

1.1 Why Chair Tai Chi Is Perfect for Seniors

The Problem with Most Exercise Programs for Older Adults

Most gyms weren't built for older adults. The equipment assumes you already have the balance of a twenty-year-old, and the classes move so fast you barely have time to check your footing. That isn't just annoying; it's discouraging. It sends a subtle message that fitness belongs to the young.

This is not just unwelcoming. It is medically counterproductive. When exercise feels inaccessible, dangerous, or humiliating, people stop doing it. And when seniors stop moving, the consequences compound quickly. Muscle mass decreases. Balance deteriorates. Joints stiffen. The risk of falls rises. Energy drops. Mood follows.

The health community has known for decades that regular, gentle physical activity is one of the most powerful interventions available for healthy aging. The challenge has never been the science. It has been designing movement practices that seniors will actually do consistently and safely.

Chair Tai Chi solves that problem.

What Makes It Different

Traditional Tai Chi, practiced standing, is already considered one of the gentlest and most accessible movement practices in the world. It originated in ancient China not as a fitness trend but as a complete system for cultivating health, balance, and inner calm through slow, flowing movement. Unlike high-impact exercise, it places no jarring stress on the joints. Unlike yoga, it requires no floor work or flexibility that most older adults do not have. Unlike walking, it can be practiced indoors in any weather, in a small space, by anyone regardless of cardiovascular fitness.

Chair Tai Chi takes all of those advantages and removes the one remaining barrier that stops many seniors from practicing: the requirement to stand.

By performing the movements from a sturdy chair, the practice becomes accessible to people who:

- Use a walker or wheelchair for some or all of their daily mobility

- Have had recent joint replacement surgery and are still in recovery

- Live with chronic conditions such as osteoporosis, arthritis, or Parkinson's disease

- Experience dizziness, vertigo, or balance disorders that make standing exercise risky

- Are simply new to exercise and lack the lower body strength or confidence to begin on their feet

- Have had a fear of falling that keeps them from engaging in any physical activity at all

This is not a watered-down version of Tai Chi. Research published in journals including the *Journal of Aging and Physical Activity* and the *British Journal of Sports Medicine* has consistently found that seated Tai Chi produces measurable improvements in balance, flexibility, pain levels, and mental health outcomes comparable to those seen in standing practice. The chair is not a limitation. For the right person, it is the tool that makes everything possible.

Adapting to Every Level of Ability

One of the most important things to understand about this program is that there is no single correct way to do any of the movements described in this book. Every exercise comes with modifications, ranging from a very small range of motion all the way to a fuller expression of the movement for those who have the capacity for it.

A person living with severe rheumatoid arthritis in both hands may practice the arm movements with loose, open palms rather than the more elaborate hand positions used in traditional Tai Chi forms. A person recovering from a hip replacement may restrict their leg movements to gentle, controlled slides of the foot along the floor rather than any kind of lift. A person with no physical limitations at all may add slow, controlled upper body rotation and deeper breathing to intensify the experience without adding any impact or risk.

All of these people are doing Chair Tai Chi. All of them are receiving its benefits. None of them is doing it wrong.

This adaptability is by design, and it reflects a core principle of both Tai Chi philosophy and modern geriatric exercise science: the goal is never performance. The goal is progress, however small, sustained over time.

Safety as a Foundation, Not an Afterthought

In over fifteen years of teaching Chair Tai Chi to seniors in community centers, assisted living facilities, and rehabilitation settings, I have witnessed almost no injuries from the practice itself. The movements are inherently safe because they are slow, controlled, and never push the body to its limit. There is no momentum to lose control of, no weight to drop, no explosive movement that could catch a joint off guard.

That said, safety in this program is treated as a foundation, not just a disclaimer at the front of the book. Every exercise has been reviewed with physical and occupational therapists. The progression across four weeks is deliberate, building gradually so that your body has time to adapt. Instructions are given not just for how to do each movement but for how to recognize when to back off, when to rest, and when to consult your healthcare provider.

The chair itself, properly chosen and properly positioned, becomes an anchor of safety. It gives your body a reference point that eliminates the cognitive load of balancing while standing, which frees your nervous system to focus entirely on the movement, the breath, and the internal experience of the practice.

We will cover chair setup in detail in Chapter 2. For now, the key point is this: Chair Tai Chi was not designed by taking a standing practice and making it easier. It was designed from the ground up for bodies that deserve a practice that respects exactly what they are and what they need.

1.2 The Mind-Body Connection

A Practice That Works From the Inside Out

Most Western exercise is built around an outside-in model. You move your body through a prescribed range of motion, you burn calories, you build muscle, and the benefits accumulate over time. The mind is largely incidental to the process. You might listen to music, watch television, or mentally run through your grocery list while riding a stationary bike, and the cardiovascular benefit will be roughly the same.

Tai Chi works differently. It is built around what Chinese medicine has always called the mind-body connection, the understanding that the quality of your attention during movement is not separate from the physical benefit of the movement. It is part of it.

In every session of this program, you will be asked to do something that sounds deceptively simple: pay attention. Notice where your hands are in space. Feel the weight of your arms. Follow the movement of your breath. Observe, without judgment, how your body feels today compared to yesterday.

This quality of attention is not just a philosophical add-on to the physical exercises. It is the mechanism by which Tai Chi produces many of its most significant benefits, particularly in the areas of stress reduction, mental clarity, and emotional regulation.

Breath as the Bridge

If there is one element that makes Chair Tai Chi fundamentally different from passive sitting or conventional stretching, it is the breath.

In Tai Chi, the breath is not an afterthought. It is the conductor of the entire practice. Every movement is coordinated with either an inhale or an exhale. Opening movements, those that expand the chest or lift the arms outward, are paired with inhalation. Closing movements, those that bring the arms inward or gently compress the front body, are paired with exhalation. Over time, this pairing becomes automatic, and the breath begins to function as a continuous, gentle massage of the nervous system.

Here is the physiology behind why that matters. The human nervous system operates on two primary tracks. The sympathetic nervous system, often called the fight-or-flight system, governs the stress response. It accelerates the heart rate, tightens the muscles, sharpens the senses, and floods the body with cortisol and adrenaline. This system is essential for survival, but in modern life, and particularly in the lives of older adults managing chronic illness, pain, financial stress, or social isolation, it tends to run at a higher baseline than is healthy.

The parasympathetic nervous system, often called the rest-and-digest system, does the opposite. It slows the heart rate, relaxes the muscles, improves digestion, and promotes the hormonal conditions associated with healing, deep sleep, and emotional calm.

Slow, diaphragmatic breathing, the kind practiced in Tai Chi, is one of the most direct and reliable ways to shift the nervous system from sympathetic dominance to parasympathetic engagement. Every long, slow exhale sends a signal through the vagus nerve that tells the body it is safe, that the crisis is over, that it can soften now.

For seniors dealing with chronic pain, anxiety, or the accumulated stress of aging, this physiological shift is not a minor side benefit. It is genuinely therapeutic. A 2021 study in *Frontiers in Psychology* found that eight weeks of mind-body practice including slow breath-synchronized movement significantly reduced cortisol levels and self-reported anxiety scores in adults over 65, with benefits that persisted at a three-month follow-up.

Mental Engagement and Cognitive Health

There is another layer to the mind-body connection in Tai Chi that deserves particular attention when we are talking about seniors: the cognitive demands of the practice.

Chair Tai Chi requires the brain to do several things at once. It asks you to track the position of your hands and arms in space (proprioception). It asks you to coordinate movement with breath timing (temporal coordination). It asks you to sequence movements in a specific order (working memory). And it asks you to do all of this while maintaining a quality of calm, focused attention (executive function and attention regulation).

None of these demands are overwhelming. That is the point. They are gently, consistently stimulating in a way that keeps the brain engaged without generating frustration or cognitive overload. Neurologists sometimes refer to this zone as the "sweet spot" for brain training, challenging enough to require effort, simple enough to allow success.

Research from the University of Illinois found that older adults who practiced mind-body movement for twelve weeks showed improvements in working memory and processing speed comparable to those seen from aerobic exercise, while also reporting significantly higher enjoyment and lower dropout rates. The enjoyment factor is not trivial. Practices that feel good are practices people sustain, and sustained practice is where real cognitive benefits accumulate.

Many students in my classes report noticeably sharper focus within the first one to two weeks. This is not imagined. The combination of increased cerebral blood flow from gentle movement, reduced cortisol from breath practice, and the cognitive engagement of learning new sequences all contribute to what feels like a kind of mental brightening. Things that felt foggy begin to come into focus. Sleep often improves. The general sense of being overwhelmed by small things gradually lightens.

Presence as Medicine

There is one more dimension of the mind-body connection worth naming here, and it is harder to quantify than cortisol levels or memory scores, but no less real.

Tai Chi is, at its heart, a practice of presence. Not the performative mindfulness of forcing yourself to feel grateful or calm, but the simple, practical act of bringing your full attention into your body, into this breath, into this moment.

For many seniors, this is more radical than it sounds. The experience of aging can bring with it a persistent backward-looking quality, grief for what the body used to be able to do, worry about what comes next, a sense of discontinuity from the person you were thirty years ago. Chair Tai Chi does not pretend these feelings do not exist. But it offers, for ten minutes a day, an anchor in the present that gradually changes the relationship between the mind and the body. The body stops being an obstacle or a source of bad news. It becomes, again, a home.

Students who have practiced for even a few weeks often describe a subtle but significant shift in how they relate to physical discomfort. Pain that was previously experienced as alarming, as a sign of danger or decline, begins to be met with more equanimity. This is not because the pain disappears. It is because the mind has been trained, gently and consistently, to observe sensation rather than react to it.

This quality of equanimous attention is one of the oldest documented benefits of Tai Chi practice, described in Chinese medical texts going back centuries, and now being increasingly validated by modern pain science, which understands that the brain's interpretation of pain signals is far more plastic than we once believed.

1.3 Health Benefits for Seniors

What the Research Says and What Students Report

The evidence base for Tai Chi as a health intervention for older adults is now one of the most robust in complementary medicine. Over the past two decades, hundreds of peer-reviewed studies have examined its effects on specific health outcomes in older populations. The findings are consistent enough that the American College of Sports Medicine, the Centers for Disease Control, and numerous national rheumatology associations now formally recommend Tai Chi as part of a healthy aging exercise program.

What follows is a detailed look at the primary health benefits documented for Chair Tai Chi specifically, along with real-world observations from students and clinical partners I have worked with across fifteen years of practice.

Improved Mobility and Flexibility

One of the most immediate and noticeable effects of Chair Tai Chi is an improvement in the range of motion available in the upper body, particularly in the shoulders, neck, and thoracic spine, areas that are commonly stiff in sedentary older adults.

The seated movements in this program take the shoulder joint through its full natural arc in multiple directions. They gently rotate the thoracic vertebrae, which tend to become rigid with age and prolonged sitting. They stretch the muscles of the chest and upper back that become chronically shortened in people who spend significant time in a forward-facing, seated posture.

For seniors with osteoarthritis, the slow, lubricated movement of the joint through its range of motion is one of the primary mechanisms of pain relief. Synovial fluid, the joint's natural lubricant, is distributed through movement. Joints that remain still become progressively stiffer and more painful. Regular, gentle movement counteracts this process without the inflammation risk that comes from higher-impact exercise.

I'll never forget a 72-year-old student in one of my classes whose surgeon gave her the news nobody wants to hear: her shoulder was 'bone on bone.' He told her she just had to accept losing her range of motion as she got older. She decided to do these exact seated movements twice a day anyway. About six weeks later, she walked into the community center and reached her arm completely over her head, without a flinch, for the first time in four years. When she went back for her next checkup, even her surgeon was surprised. The slow, gentle motion had naturally coaxed her body into lubricating the joint again.

This is not a miraculous outcome. It is the predictable result of appropriate, consistent movement applied to a joint that had been deprived of it.

Better Balance and Fall Prevention

Falls are the leading cause of injury-related death in adults over 65 in the United States, according to the Centers for Disease Control and Prevention. Each year, approximately 36 million falls occur among older Americans, resulting in 32,000 deaths and over 300,000 hospitalizations for hip fractures alone. The fear of falling is itself a significant health problem, causing many older adults to restrict their activity to a degree that accelerates the very physical decline that makes falls more likely.

Tai Chi has more high-quality evidence supporting its effectiveness as a fall prevention intervention than almost any other exercise modality. A landmark meta-analysis published in the *Journal of the American Geriatrics Society* found that Tai Chi reduced the rate of falls in community-dwelling older adults by 43 to 50 percent, an effect size that no pharmaceutical intervention has matched.

Chair Tai Chi improves balance through several distinct mechanisms. First, the seated movements train proprioception, the body's internal sense of where its parts are in space, which is a primary component of balance that declines with age. Second, the program progressively strengthens the core muscles, the deep abdominals and spinal stabilizers, that are the foundation of postural stability in any position. Third, the practice includes specific movements that challenge and train the vestibular system, the inner ear's balance apparatus, in a controlled, safe environment where the consequences of a moment of instability are minimal.

Fourth, and perhaps most importantly for the large number of seniors whose fall risk is increased by fear, Chair Tai Chi builds a quality of embodied confidence that transfers to standing and walking. Students who have spent weeks learning to move their bodies with precision and intentionality begin to move through the world differently. They walk more deliberately. They are more aware of their footing. They respond to unexpected shifts in balance with less panic and more coordination.

Cardiovascular Health and Circulation

Chair Tai Chi is a low-intensity aerobic activity, which means it elevates heart rate modestly while providing the circulation-improving benefits of sustained movement. For seniors who cannot perform moderate-intensity aerobic exercise, this represents a meaningful alternative that is almost universally accessible.

The continuous, flowing movements of the practice require a sustained increase in peripheral circulation, meaning that more blood is delivered to the muscles and extremities than at complete rest. For seniors with poor circulation, cold hands and feet, or peripheral vascular disease, even this modest increase in blood flow can produce noticeable improvements in comfort and sensation.

The deep diaphragmatic breathing that accompanies every movement has its own cardiovascular benefit. Each full breath cycle creates a slight change in intrathoracic pressure that acts as an auxiliary pump for the venous return of blood to the heart. Over the course of a ten-minute session, hundreds of these micro-pumping actions contribute to improved circulation throughout the entire system.

Joint Health and Arthritis Management

Arthritis, in its various forms, affects more than 54 million American adults, and prevalence increases dramatically with age. By age 65, roughly half of all adults have been diagnosed with some form of arthritis, making it one of the most significant barriers to physical activity in the senior population.

The design of Chair Tai Chi movements makes them particularly well-suited to arthritic bodies. There is no jarring impact, no position that requires the joint to bear excessive load, and no movement that goes to the end range of motion where arthritic joints experience the most pain and instability. The movements stay in the comfortable middle range where the joint can function smoothly.

For rheumatoid arthritis specifically, the anti-inflammatory effect of regular, gentle movement combined with the cortisol-reducing effect of the breath practice creates a physiological environment less conducive to inflammatory flares. Several rheumatologists I have collaborated with over the years now routinely recommend Chair Tai Chi to patients as a complement to medical management, noting that patients who practice consistently tend to require lower doses of anti-inflammatory medication and report higher quality-of-life scores.

Anxiety Reduction and Emotional Regulation

The mental health benefits of Chair Tai Chi are, in my experience, often the most profound for the students who need it most. And the need is significant. Depression affects an estimated 7 million Americans over age 65, while anxiety disorders affect a similar number. Both conditions are frequently underdiagnosed and undertreated in older adults, who may minimize their symptoms, attribute them to normal aging, or face barriers to accessing mental health care.

The mechanisms by which Tai Chi reduces anxiety are now fairly well understood. The breath-synchronized movement activates the parasympathetic nervous system, as described earlier. The rhythmic, repetitive nature of the movements has an almost meditative effect on the mind, interrupting the cycle of ruminative thinking that drives both anxiety and depression. The gradual experience of mastery, of learning movements, remembering sequences, and noticing improvement over time, builds a sense of self-efficacy that directly counters the helplessness that often accompanies chronic illness or functional decline.

For many older adults, there is also something deeply meaningful about dedicating time each day to their own wellness. In a life stage where the cultural narrative often frames the elderly as recipients of care rather than agents of their own health, a daily practice that says 'I am taking care of myself' can change the way a person carries themselves through the rest of the day. I've seen it happen hundreds of times.

Cognitive Function and Mental Clarity

The relationship between regular gentle exercise and cognitive health in older adults has been one of the most active areas of geroscience research over the past decade. The evidence increasingly supports the idea that movement, particularly mind-body movement that engages attention and coordination, is one of the most effective tools available for slowing cognitive decline and potentially reducing the risk of dementia.

Tai Chi practice increases cerebral blood flow, which improves the delivery of oxygen and glucose to brain cells. It stimulates the production of brain-derived neurotrophic factor (BDNF), a protein that supports the growth and maintenance of neurons and is associated with improved learning and memory. It engages the prefrontal cortex, hippocampus, and cerebellum, brain regions associated with executive function, spatial memory, and motor coordination respectively, in a way that few other activities do simultaneously.

A study from Harvard Medical School found that older adults who practiced Tai Chi twice weekly for twelve weeks showed significant improvements in cognitive assessments measuring attention, processing speed, and executive function, as well as increases in gray matter volume in brain regions associated with these functions. Notably, the improvements were most pronounced in participants who had shown early signs of cognitive decline at the start of the study, suggesting that Tai Chi may be particularly valuable as an early intervention for cognitive aging.

Students in my classes frequently report improvements in mental clarity after one to two weeks of consistent practice. Descriptions range from "the fog lifted a bit" to "I remembered three things I had been forgetting for months." These subjective reports are consistent with what the research measures objectively and they matter, because the subjective experience of mental sharpness has an enormous impact on quality of life, confidence, and independence.

Sleep Quality

Though often overlooked in discussions of exercise benefits for seniors, improved sleep quality is one of the most consistently reported outcomes of Tai Chi practice, and one of the most impactful for overall health.

Poor sleep is epidemic among older adults. Changes in circadian rhythm, reduced production of melatonin, increased nighttime pain, anxiety, and the side effects of multiple medications all contribute to the widely reported experience among seniors of lying awake for hours, waking frequently, or never feeling truly rested even after a full night in bed.

Chair Tai Chi addresses sleep quality through multiple pathways. The reduction in cortisol levels makes the transition into sleep physiologically easier. The parasympathetic activation produced by breath-focused movement trains the nervous system to access a state of calm that is the necessary precursor to sleep onset. The physical benefit of having moved the body gently during the day contributes to what sleep researchers call "sleep drive," the biological pressure to rest that builds throughout the day and facilitates both falling asleep and staying asleep.

Several students have told me, in remarkably similar language, that they started the program hoping to improve their flexibility and ended up most grateful for the fact that they finally started sleeping through the night.

A Note on Individual Results

Every benefit described in this chapter is well-supported by research and observed consistently across thousands of students. But it is also true that individual results vary. The pace at which you notice improvement will depend on your starting point, your consistency, your specific health conditions, and factors as personal as your stress levels and the quality of your diet.

What I can promise you, with confidence built from fifteen years of watching people transform through this practice, is this: if you show up for ten minutes a day over the next four weeks and follow this program with genuine attention, you will feel different at the end than you do right now. Not miraculously different. Not dramatically different overnight. But genuinely, measurably, sustainably different in ways that will matter to your daily life.

That is worth showing up for.

The next chapter will prepare you practically for the work ahead, covering everything you need to know about setting up your space, choosing the right chair, understanding safety guidelines, and beginning your first session with confidence.

Chapter 2: Preparing for Chair Tai Chi

Starting something new takes courage, especially when your body has been through changes that make you more cautious than you once were. Maybe you've tried exercise programs before that felt too fast, too hard, or too disconnected from where you actually are physically. Maybe a doctor or family member suggested this, and part of you is still not sure you're the "exercise type." Maybe you are eager and ready and simply want to know what to do next.

Wherever you are starting from, this chapter is for you.

Preparation in Chair Tai Chi is not just logistical. It is an act of care toward yourself. Choosing the right chair, creating a space that feels inviting, understanding the basic safety principles, and approaching your practice with the right mental posture are not preliminary steps before the real work begins. They are the real work. They are the difference between a practice that lasts four weeks and one that becomes part of your life.

Let's walk through each piece carefully, because you deserve to begin this program with everything set up properly in your favor.

2.1 Choosing the Right Chair

Why the Chair Matters More Than You Might Think

In most fitness programs, equipment is secondary. In Chair Tai Chi, the chair is central. It is your foundation, your anchor, and the tool that makes every movement possible. A poorly chosen chair can create discomfort, promote poor posture, limit your range of motion, or, in the worst case, compromise your stability during practice. A well-chosen chair does the opposite. It quietly supports every movement you make, freeing your attention from physical uncertainty and directing it toward the practice itself.

This is not a place to cut corners, and fortunately it is also not a place that requires spending money. The right chair for Chair Tai Chi is most likely already in your home.

The Characteristics of an Ideal Chair

Your chair is your most important tool. You don't need to buy anything fancy. In fact, your dining room chair is probably perfect, but you do need to be picky. If your chair wobbles, you'll spend your energy worrying about falling instead of focusing on your breath. Here's what to look for:

Stability. This is the most important characteristic. Your chair must not rock, tip, wobble, or shift when you move your arms, rotate your torso, or shift your weight side to side. Four-legged chairs with a wide base are the most stable option. Avoid any chair with wheels, even if the wheels have locks. Avoid folding chairs unless they are specifically designed as heavy-duty and have been tested for stability. Avoid swivel chairs entirely. A sturdy wooden or metal dining chair is often the ideal choice.

Seat firmness. The seat surface should be firm enough to allow you to feel your sit bones, the two bony protrusions at the base of your pelvis, making contact with it. If the cushioning is so soft that you sink significantly into the seat, your pelvis will tilt backward, rounding your lower back and collapsing your posture. This not only limits the quality of your movement but can contribute to lower back strain over time. If your preferred chair has a very soft cushion, consider placing a thin, firm pillow or folded blanket on the seat to raise and firm the surface.

Seat height. When you sit toward the front half of the seat with your feet flat on the floor, your knees should form approximately a 90-degree angle. Your thighs should be roughly parallel to the ground or angled very slightly downward toward the knees. If the chair is too low, your knees will be higher than your hips, which compresses the hip flexors and makes upright posture significantly harder to maintain. If the chair is too high, your feet may dangle, which removes the grounding that proper practice requires.

To adjust for height, use a firm, non-slip footrest if the chair is too tall for your leg length. If the chair seat is too low, a firm seat cushion of two to four inches can raise your sitting height effectively. The key is that your feet must be fully supported by either the floor or a stable footrest throughout every practice session.

Back support. Your chair should have a backrest that supports a neutral, upright spinal position. A straight or very slightly angled backrest is ideal. Chairs with heavily reclined backrests, pronounced lumbar curves, or bucket seats that angle the pelvis backward will work against the upright posture that Tai Chi requires. That said, you do not need to rest against the backrest during practice. In most movements, you will sit a few inches away from the back of the chair, upright and self-supported. The backrest is there as a reference and a reassurance, not as a constant support.

Armrests. Armrests are useful for stability during transitions and can provide confidence for those who feel less secure in seated positions. However, armrests should not limit your ability to move your arms freely through the movements. If the armrests are very high, very wide, or positioned in a way that your arms hit them during side or forward movements, they become an obstacle rather than a help. Test this before your first session by slowly sweeping your arms in the basic directions of the practice movements. If the armrests interfere, an armless chair is a better choice.

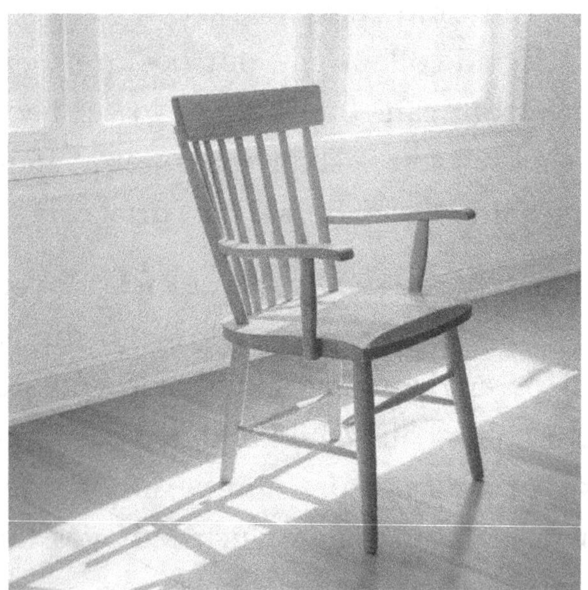

The Ideal Practice Chair – Armrest

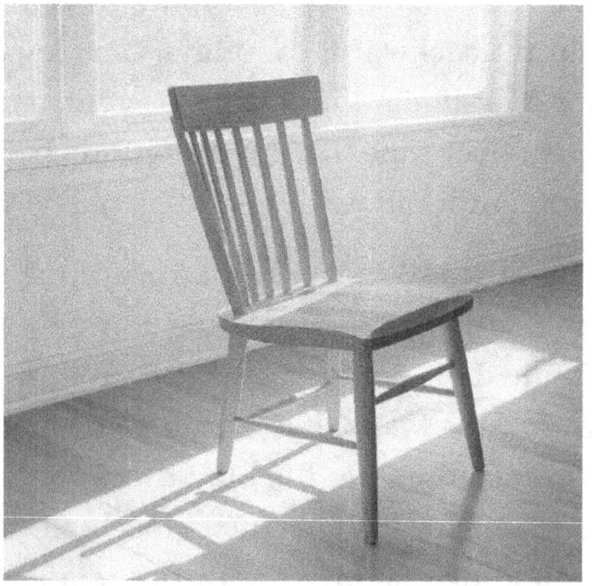

The Ideal Practice Chair – Armless

Testing Your Chair Before You Begin

Once you have identified your chair, perform this simple stability and comfort check before your first practice session.

Step 1: Sit toward the front half of the seat, feet flat on the floor, hip-width apart. Notice whether your feet are fully supported.

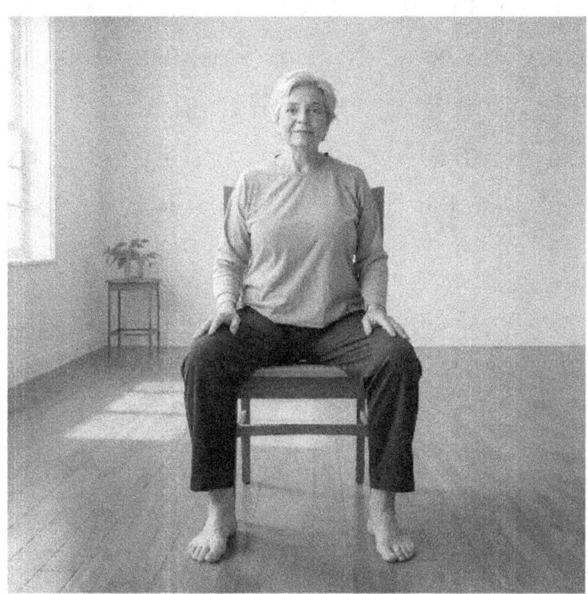

Step 2: Press gently but firmly into the chair with both hands on the sides of the seat and rock your weight subtly side to side. The chair should feel completely immovable.

Step 3: Raise both arms slowly out to your sides and forward, mimicking a gentle sweeping movement. Check that no part of the chair blocks the motion.

Step 4: Gently rotate your upper body a few degrees to the right and then to the left. The chair should remain fully stable throughout. If it passes all three checks, you have found your practice chair.

A Note on Placement

Position your chair on a firm, level surface. Avoid thick rugs or uneven flooring. If your home has mostly thick carpet and a harder floor is not available, place a non-slip mat beneath the chair legs to prevent any sliding during practice. Ensure there is at least two to three feet of clear space on either side of the chair and in front of it, and at least one foot of clearance behind the backrest.

2.2 Setting Up Your Practice Space

The Environment Is Part of the Practice

Tai Chi is really a practice of paying attention. Everything about it; the movement, the breath, even the space you practice in, is designed to sharpen your awareness. The quality of your sensory environment during those ten minutes has a direct effect on how easily you can access that awareness. A cluttered, noisy, or poorly lit space creates mental friction that you will then have to work against every time you sit down to practice. A calm, organized, and inviting space does the opposite. It primes your nervous system for the kind of attentive relaxation that makes Chair Tai Chi most effective.

Setting up your practice space does not require redecorating a room. It requires making a series of small, deliberate choices about how you use an existing space in your home.

Flooring and Physical Safety

The floor around your practice area matters for two reasons: it affects the stability of your chair, and it affects what happens on the rare occasion that you need to stand, step, or reach for something.

Hardwood, laminate, tile, and low-pile carpet are all suitable surfaces. Thick, plush carpet or area rugs that might bunch or shift are less ideal. If you practice on a smooth hard floor, make sure the chair legs have rubber feet or non-slip pads to prevent sliding.

Remove any portable rugs, mats, electrical cords, pet toys, low furniture, or other objects from the immediate area around your chair before each session. You do not need a large clear area, just enough that if you lean slightly or extend an arm or leg, you will not contact anything unexpected.

Lighting

Natural light is ideal for morning or midday practice. Position your chair to take advantage of any available natural light, ideally facing toward or beside a window rather than directly into the sun. Natural light supports alertness, elevates mood, and creates a sense of connection to the environment outside that many students find gently energizing.

For evening practice or in rooms with limited natural light, use warm, ambient lighting rather than harsh overhead fluorescents. The goal is enough light to practice comfortably, see your hands and feet clearly, and remain mentally alert, without the visual harshness that makes relaxation difficult. Dimmer switches, floor lamps, or side table lamps on a warm setting work well.

Avoid practicing in very dim or dark conditions. This is both a safety consideration and a practical one. Your visual system contributes significantly to your sense of spatial orientation and balance, and practicing in good light keeps all of your sensory input working in harmony.

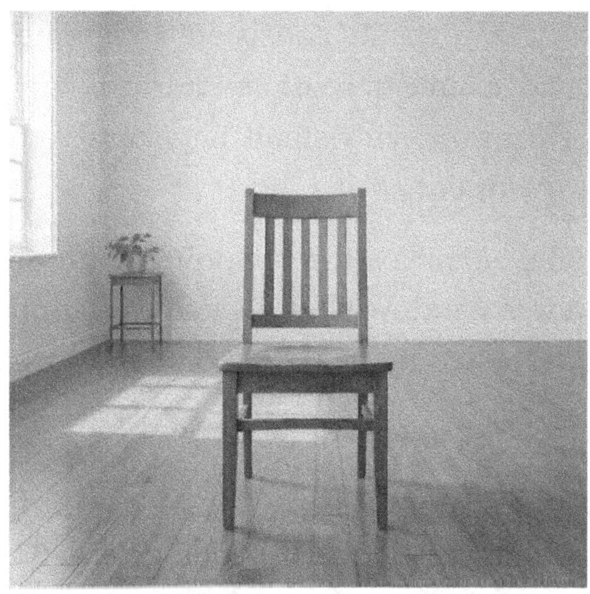

The Practice Space Setup

Sound Environment

Silence is optimal, especially in the early weeks when you are learning movement sequences and working to maintain focused attention. Even familiar background noise, a television on in another room, a radio playing, or background conversation, creates competition for your attention that you will not notice until you practice without it and realize how much calmer the experience feels.

If complete quiet is not available in your home, try using soft instrumental music without lyrics. Traditional Chinese instrumental music is a classic choice and is widely available through streaming services. Soft nature sounds, gentle classical music, or ambient soundscapes also work well. The key is that the audio should require no active listening. It should sit in the background and soften the sonic environment, not engage your mind.

Turn off or silence your mobile phone before each session. If you use a timer, set it before you begin and place the phone face-down. The ten minutes you spend on this practice are yours, and they deserve the same protected attention you would give a medical appointment or a meal you actually want to enjoy.

Temperature and Air Quality

Practice in a room with comfortable, consistent temperature. Cold muscles are stiffer and more prone to discomfort, so if your home is cool, consider a light layer of clothing or a brief warm-up with small hand and wrist movements before beginning the session's main sequence.

Fresh air, when available, enhances the breathing component of the practice. If weather permits, cracking a window slightly creates a subtle freshness that many practitioners find conducive to a more alert and clear-headed session.

Creating Consistency in Your Space

Practicing in the same physical location every day, or at least as consistently as possible, contributes to what behavioral psychologists call environmental cueing. Your brain begins to associate a specific physical context with a specific mental and physical state. Over time, walking to your practice chair and sitting down begins to automatically trigger a shift toward the relaxed alertness that your sessions require, before you have even taken your first breath.

This is not mystical. It is the same mechanism that makes you feel sleepy when you lie in your bed, or hungry when you sit at your kitchen table. Environments trigger states. Build the association intentionally, and your practice will become progressively easier to drop into regardless of how your day is going.

Even small, consistent details help. Placing your practice chair in the same spot each time, using the same light source, keeping a glass of water nearby in the same cup, these small repetitions reinforce the environmental cue and deepen the association over time.

2.3 Safety First

Safety Is Not a Warning. It Is a Practice.

I used to rush through the safety talk in my classes because I wanted to get to the 'fun stuff.' I was wrong. I quickly learned that safety is the practice. Moving carefully isn't about being fearful; it's about treating your body with the respect it has earned.

Both require awareness. Both require honesty about your current state. Both require the willingness to move more slowly than you feel you need to, until you know your body's responses well enough to make informed choices about pace and range. When you approach safety in this spirit, it stops feeling like a list of restrictions and begins to feel like self-respect in action.

Preparing Your Environment Before Each Session

Before every practice session, take ninety seconds to check your environment. This is not a suggestion for beginners only. It is a habit that experienced practitioners maintain throughout their years of practice, because environments change and attention to them never becomes unnecessary.

Walk the area around your practice chair and clear anything that was not there last time: a bag set down after shopping, a pet that has settled near the chair, a glass of water on the floor nearby, or any other object that occupies the space where your feet or body might move. Confirm that the chair has not shifted since you last used it and that it remains on a stable surface.

Check that your footwear is appropriate. For Chair Tai Chi practice, flat, closed-toe shoes with non-slip soles are ideal. Well-fitted athletic shoes or sturdy flats with rubber soles work well. Avoid high heels, loose slippers, open-back sandals, or any footwear that might slip off your foot or fail to grip the floor firmly. If you prefer to practice in socks, choose socks with non-slip grip on the soles, which are widely available and specifically designed for activities where stability matters.

Physical Safety During Practice

The movements in this program are designed to stay well within your comfortable range of motion. You should never feel pain during any exercise in this book. Mild muscle awareness, that gentle confirmation that a muscle has been gently engaged or a joint has been moved through its range, is normal and healthy. Sharp pain, joint pain, chest pain, dizziness, shortness of breath, or any sensation that feels wrong is a signal to stop immediately.

When you stop, rest in your chair. Breathe slowly. If the sensation passes quickly and you can identify its cause, such as moving too far or too fast in a particular direction, you can resume practice with smaller, more careful movements. If the sensation does not pass, if you feel any chest discomfort, unusual shortness of breath, severe dizziness, or sharp radiating pain anywhere in the body, stop for the day and contact your healthcare provider before the next session.

Do not practice immediately after a large meal. Give yourself at least ninety minutes between eating and practice to allow digestion to settle and to ensure comfortable deep breathing.

If you have had recent surgery, a recent fall, an acute injury flare, or a period of illness, hold off on practice until you have been medically cleared. Chair Tai Chi is gentle enough to be appropriate for most physical conditions, but "gentle" is not the same as "appropriate for every situation without any consultation."

Working with Your Healthcare Team

Many students come to Chair Tai Chi on the recommendation of their physician, physical therapist, or occupational therapist, and this collaboration is genuinely valuable. If you have a regular healthcare provider, consider mentioning that you are beginning this program. Most will be encouraging, and some may have specific recommendations based on your individual health history.

If you have specific physical conditions that affect your movement, such as vertebral compression fractures, severe osteoporosis, recent cardiac events, uncontrolled blood pressure, or neurological conditions, consult your provider before beginning. In most cases the answer will be a modified form of practice rather than avoidance, but getting that guidance first is the responsible and empowering choice.

Physical therapists in particular are excellent allies for Chair Tai Chi practitioners. If you currently work with a physical therapist, show them this book. Many PTs are familiar with Tai Chi as a rehabilitative practice and can help you adapt specific movements to your particular needs.

The Chair as Your Safety Anchor

One of the most important safety features of this practice is the one that is always right there with you: the chair. During any movement where you feel uncertain, you can press your palms gently onto the chair armrests or seat surface to re-establish your sense of grounding. During any movement involving the upper body, both feet remain flat on the floor and both sit bones remain in contact with the seat, providing a stable, three-point base.

In the standing version of Tai Chi, maintaining balance is an active physical effort that requires constant micro-adjustments. In Chair Tai Chi, the chair absorbs that effort entirely, which is why the practice is simultaneously more accessible for people with balance challenges and more focused for everyone else. Your body's energy is redirected from the work of not falling toward the work of moving well.

Internalize this early: the chair is not a sign that you are not strong enough to stand. The chair is the tool that makes every movement cleaner, more controlled, and more deeply felt.

2.4 Preparing Mentally for Practice

The Moment Before You Begin

There is a particular moment that good Tai Chi teachers cultivate in their students, and it happens before the first movement of every session. It is the moment of arrival. The transition from being someone who is about to practice to someone who is already present in practice.

Most of us arrive at any activity still carrying the cognitive residue of whatever came before. The unresolved conversation from this morning, the task you keep meaning to do, the worry that surfaces without warning and takes up space in the back of your awareness. These are not problems to solve before you can practice. They are simply the natural content of a full human mind. Preparing mentally for Chair Tai Chi does not mean emptying your mind of all of that. It means learning to set it aside intentionally, the way you might set down a bag when you sit at a table, knowing it will be there to pick up again when you need it.

Setting an Intention

One of the most practical and effective tools for mental preparation is setting a simple intention at the start of each session. An intention in this context is not a goal or a performance target. It is a quality of attention or engagement that you want to bring to the next ten minutes.

Intentions work best when they are brief, specific to how you feel today, and entirely within your control. Here are examples of intentions that have served my students well over the years:

- "I will move as slowly as my breath allows."
- "I will notice where I am holding tension and let it soften."
- "I will be patient with myself when a movement feels unfamiliar."
- "I will give these ten minutes fully to this practice."
- "I will treat my body with kindness today."

You do not need to write your intention down, though some students find that helpful. You simply state it quietly to yourself, or even just form it clearly as a thought, at the beginning of the session. This small act of intentional framing has a measurable effect on the quality of practice that follows, because it shifts your orientation from passive participation to active, purposeful engagement.

Patience: The Most Important Quality You Bring

Tai Chi is not a practice where effort produces results in proportion to its intensity. In fact, the relationship works almost in reverse. The more forcefully you try to move, the more tension you introduce into the movement, and the less effectively Tai Chi's benefits are delivered. The softer, slower, and more patient your approach, the more deeply the practice reaches.

This runs counter to the ethos of most Western exercise, which is built around the premise that harder is better. Learning to find quality in gentleness is one of the first and most rewarding lessons Chair Tai Chi teaches, and it is, for many students, one that translates meaningfully into how they approach other aspects of their lives.

Give yourself permission to be a beginner. Give yourself permission to move imperfectly. In the first weeks of this program, focus on familiarity with the movements, not mastery of them. If a movement takes two weeks to feel natural, that is not slow progress. That is exactly the right pace.

Many students tell me that the first week of practice felt awkward, and that by the third week they could not imagine having stopped. The students who made it to the third week were simply the ones who kept showing up without demanding that they be further along than they were.

Staying Present During Practice

The quality of attention you bring to each movement is what separates Chair Tai Chi from passive stretching or mechanical exercise repetition. When you move with genuine awareness, feeling the weight of your arm, noticing the length of your exhale, observing the subtle sensation of rotation in your spine, the practice becomes something alive. When the mind wanders and the body moves on autopilot, the movements may still be happening, but much of what makes Tai Chi uniquely beneficial is lost.

Staying present does not require extraordinary mental discipline. It requires a simple, repeatable strategy for returning attention when it drifts. Here are approaches that work well for different types of learners.

Breath awareness. The easiest and most reliable anchor for present-moment attention is the breath. Whenever you notice your mind has wandered, return your focus to the sensation of air entering your nostrils, filling your lungs, and slowly releasing. From that moment of breath awareness, let the movement re-emerge.

Hand awareness. During arm movements in particular, focusing attention on the sensation in your hands, their warmth, their weight, the tingling that sometimes develops as circulation improves, is a highly effective way to stay grounded in the immediate physical experience of practice.

Counting breath cycles. Some students find that counting quietly is helpful in the early weeks when movement sequences are not yet automatic. Count each exhale, from one to ten, then start again. This gives the analytical mind something simple to do while the rest of your attention softens into the movement.

Gentle eye focus. In traditional Tai Chi, gaze direction is part of the practice. For Chair Tai Chi, a simple and effective approach is to let the eyes rest with a soft, unfocused gaze about six to ten feet in front of you, level with the horizon. This slightly unfocused "soft gaze" is associated with the same parasympathetic nervous system shift as deep breathing and is used in many contemplative practices as a tool for calming mental activity.

The Close of Every Session

How you end a practice session matters as much as how you begin it. Rushing immediately from your chair into the next item on the day's agenda closes the session without allowing its effects to settle.

After your final movement of each session, take a full breath cycle in through the nose and out through the mouth. Let your hands rest comfortably in your lap. For thirty to sixty seconds, simply sit and notice. What do your hands feel like? Are your shoulders looser than when you began? Is your breathing slower? Is there any sensation of warmth or tingling in the arms, hands, or spine?

These observations are not performance metrics. They are the conversation your body is having with you, and learning to hear it is part of what Chair Tai Chi develops over time. The students who become most attuned to their bodies through this practice are the ones who give themselves those quiet moments of noticing, both at the close of sessions and gradually throughout their daily lives.

Stand up slowly, especially in the first few weeks. Take a moment in the seated position before rising, allow yourself to be aware of the transition, and push up using the chair armrests if available. There is no hurry. The practice ends when it ends, not when the timer goes off.

You are now prepared to begin.

Chapter 3: Seated Tai Chi Fundamentals

Every skilled practice has a foundation. In architecture, it is the ground beneath the structure. In music, it is the ability to hold rhythm before adding melody. In Chair Tai Chi, the foundation is three things working together: breath, posture, and basic movement. Master these three, even partially, even imperfectly, and everything else in this program will arrive more naturally and feel more rewarding.

This chapter is not about performing Tai Chi. It is about understanding it from the inside out, understanding what your breath is doing and why, what your spine is doing and why, and what happens when you move a limb with genuine slowness and intention rather than simply going through the motions. Take your time with this chapter. Read it once to familiarize yourself, then return to it as a reference during your first week of practice.

3.1 Proper Breathing Techniques

Why Breath Comes First

In most conventional exercise programs, breathing is an afterthought. In Chair Tai Chi, the breath is not incidental to the movement. In many ways, the breath is the movement, and the arms, torso, and legs are simply expressing what the breath is already doing.

When you breathe in a shallow, rapid, irregular way, your body interprets it as a signal of stress. Stress hormones increase. Muscles tighten. When you breathe slowly and fully, the opposite occurs. The entire system, muscular, neural, emotional, begins to soften and open.

Every movement sequence in this program is built around the breath. This means your first practice in Tai Chi is not learning to move. It is learning to breathe well.

Diaphragmatic Breathing: The Foundation

We're going to relearn how to breathe. Most of us breathe shallowly, up in our chest, especially when we're stressed. In Tai Chi, we breathe deep into the belly. Think of it like filling a balloon from the bottom up. This isn't just technique; it's a signal to your nervous system that you are safe.

Step 1: Sit upright in your practice chair. Place one hand flat on your chest and one hand flat on your lower abdomen just below the navel.

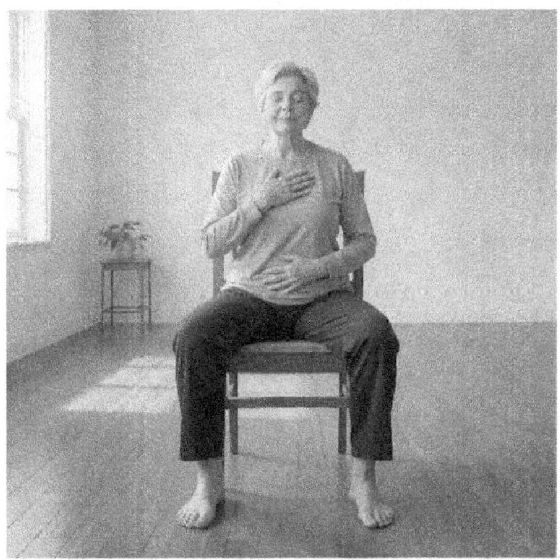

Step 2: Breathe in slowly through your nose. Direct the breath downward as though filling the bottom of your lungs first. The hand on your abdomen should rise gently outward. The hand on your chest should remain relatively still.

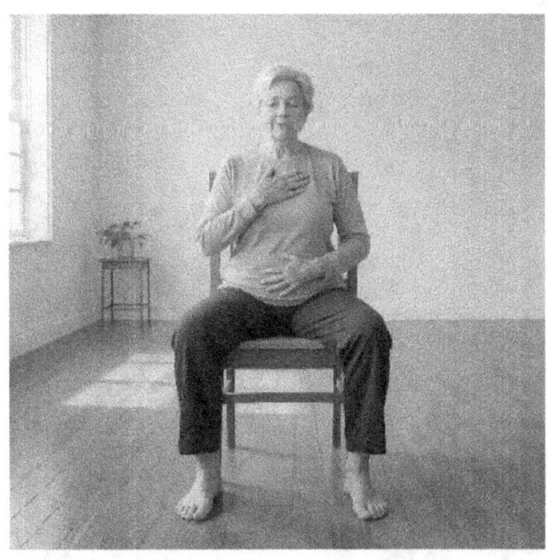

Step 3: Exhale slowly through your mouth. Allow the abdomen to soften inward as the breath releases. Let the exhale be completely passive, no pushing or forcing, simply releasing.

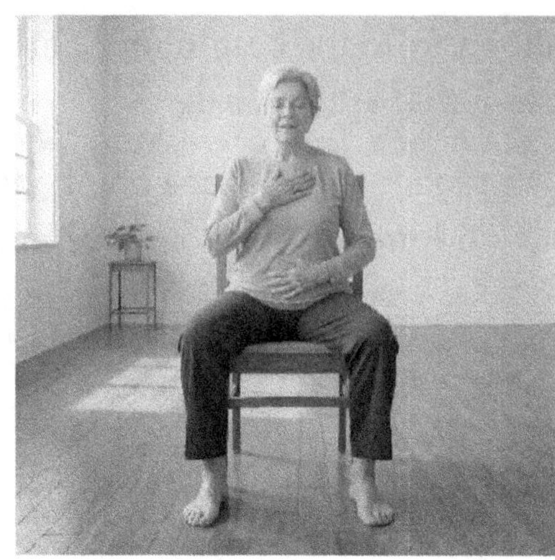

Step 4: Repeat this cycle five to six times, focusing entirely on the sensation of the abdomen rising and falling.

Coordinating Breath with Movement

Once diaphragmatic breathing feels accessible, pair it with movement. The rule in Chair Tai Chi is consistent and intuitive: **opening movements pair with inhalation, closing movements pair with exhalation.**

A simple example: slowly raise both arms from your lap out to your sides and overhead while inhaling

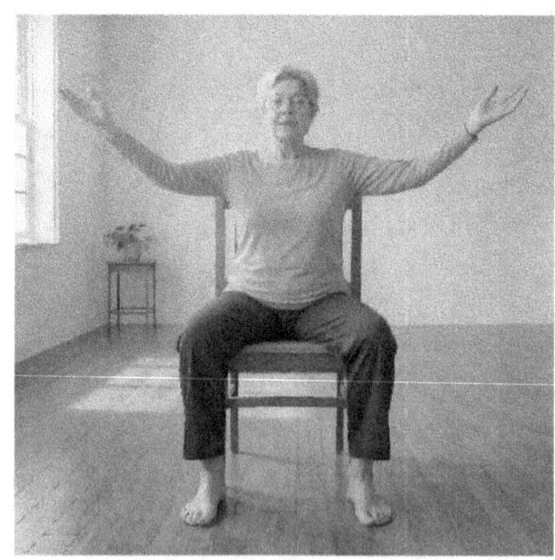

Slowly lower them back to your lap while exhaling. The inhalation seems to lift the arms. The exhalation seems to guide them back down.

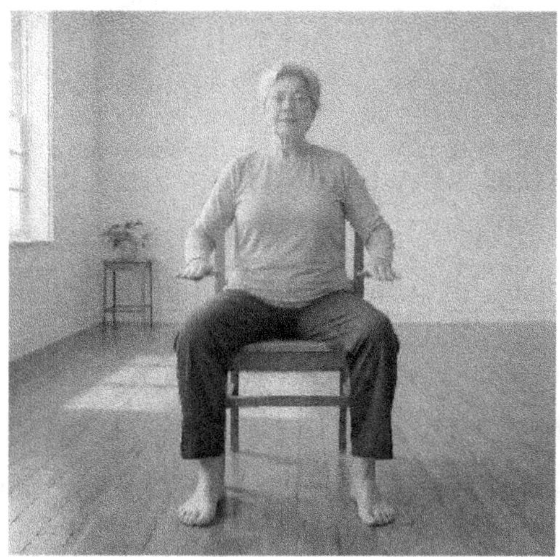

Practice this simple arm lift and lower three times before attempting any other movement in this chapter. The movement should always wait for the breath, not the other way around.

The Exhale as the Key to Relaxation

During exhalation, the parasympathetic nervous system takes over and the body measurably relaxes. Make your exhale at least as long as your inhale, and ideally slightly longer. If you inhale for a count of four, exhale for a count of five or six.

3.2 Seated Posture and Alignment

Posture as the Architecture of Movement

Good seated posture in Tai Chi is not rigid or strained. It is organized, meaning all of the body's segments are stacked in a relationship that allows weight to transfer naturally, muscles to work without overcompensating, and breathe to move freely.

The Elements of Correct Seated Posture

The sit bones and pelvis: Sit toward the front half of your chair seat. Feel the two sit bones making equal, grounded contact with the seat. From this grounding, your spine can rise naturally upward.

The spine: Imagine a thread attached to the very crown of your head, gently drawing the top of your skull upward toward the ceiling. The spine lengthens. The chest opens slightly. The lower back settles into its natural curve.

The shoulders: Let the shoulders drop away from the ears. At the start of every session and at any moment during practice when you notice the shoulders creeping upward, use the exhale to release them back down.

The hands and arms: At rest, let your hands lie loosely in your lap. Fingers are neither clenched nor stiffly extended, simply loose.

The feet: Both feet rest flat on the floor, hip-width apart. Weight is distributed evenly across the entire foot.

The head and gaze: The head sits balanced atop the spine, chin neither tucked sharply nor lifted aggressively. The gaze is directed forward with a soft, slightly unfocused quality.

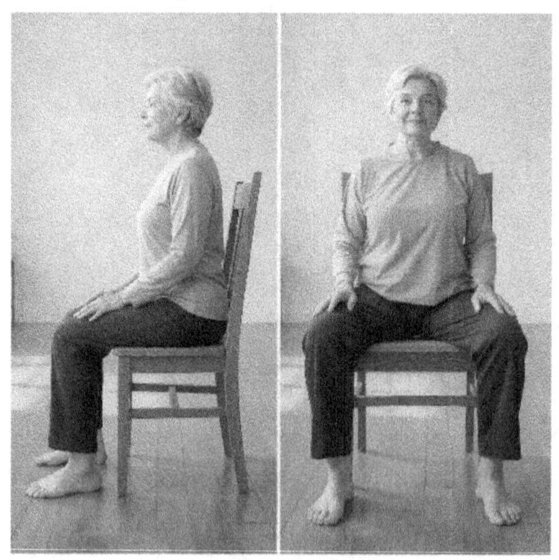

Correct Seated Posture

Good Posture vs. Common Postural Mistakes

Rounded lower back: The pelvis tilts backward, the lower back rounds, the chest collapses. Correction: roll the pelvis forward until sit bones make firm, even contact with the seat.

Excessive lower back arch: The pelvis tips too far forward. Correction: draw the lower abdomen gently inward and upward.

Elevated and tense shoulders: Shoulders pulled upward toward the ears. Correction: use the exhale to release, or exaggerate the shrug, hold two seconds, then release completely.

Forward head posture: Head juts forward beyond the shoulder line. Correction: gently draw the chin back until the back of the neck lengthens.

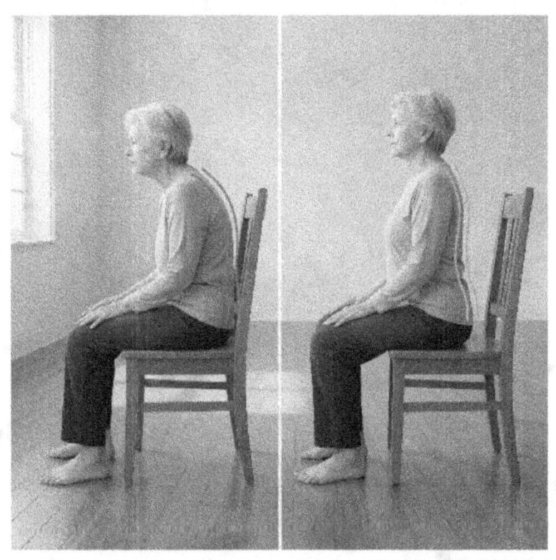

Poop Posture   Correct Posture

3.3 Basic Movements: Arm Swings, Leg Extensions, and Reaches

Moving With Intention

The three foundational movements in this section form the building blocks of every exercise sequence in the four-week program ahead. Before attempting any movement, re-establish your breath and posture as described in Sections 3.1 and 3.2.

3.3.1 Exercise 1: Gentle Arm Swings

Purpose: To warm up the shoulder joints, loosen the upper back muscles, improve arm circulation, and establish the fundamental coordination of breath with movement.

Starting position: Sit upright, feet flat on the floor hip-width apart, hands resting loosely in lap, palms facing down, shoulders relaxed.

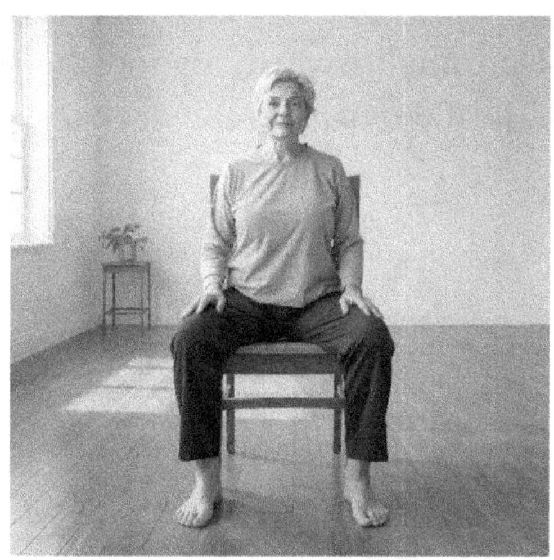

Step 1: Root and Breathe

Settle your weight evenly into the chair. Feel both sit bones grounded. Take one full diaphragmatic breath before beginning any movement.

Step 2: Float the Arms Forward

On your inhale, slowly float both arms forward and upward from the lap, leading with the back of the wrists. Allow the arms to rise to approximately shoulder height, elbows soft and slightly bent.

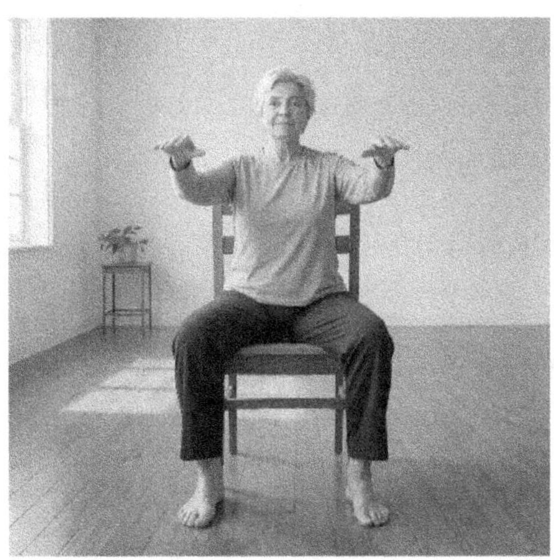

Step 3: Open and Expand

At the top of the inhale with arms at shoulder height, pause for one natural moment. Feel the gentle expansion across the chest and openness through the shoulders.

Step 4: Lower on the Exhale

As you exhale, slowly allow the arms to float back down toward the lap, palms facing downward as though gently pressing the air beneath them. Arms settle back into the lap only when the exhale is complete.

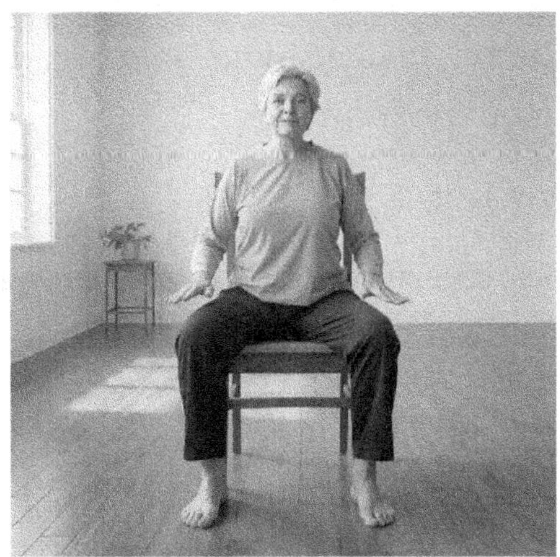

Repetitions: Four to six full cycles per session.

Modification: If raising the arms to shoulder height causes discomfort, limit the float to two to three inches from the lap. The breath-movement coordination benefit is preserved at any range.

3.3.2 Exercise 2: Seated Leg Extensions

Purpose: To activate the quadriceps and hip flexors, improve knee joint mobility, stimulate circulation in the lower limbs, and build gentle leg strength.

Starting position: Sit upright, slightly forward on the seat. Hands rest on thighs or armrests for light support.

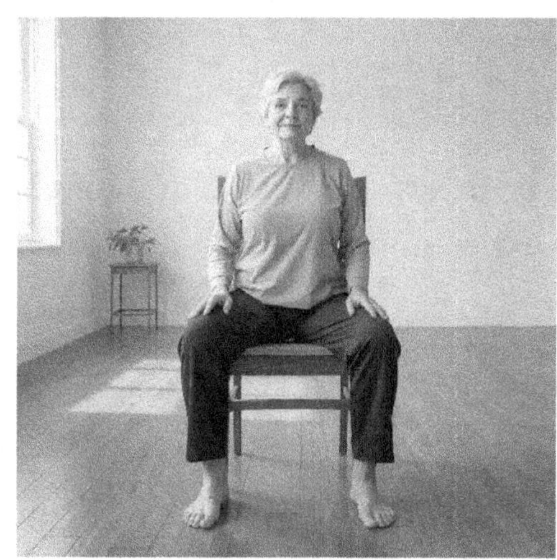

Step 1: Root and Prepare
Ground both feet into the floor. Take a single slow breath cycle. Notice the weight of both legs resting on the chair.

Step 2: Slide and Float One Leg

On your inhale, slowly slide the right foot forward along the floor, extending the right leg out in front of you. Gently flex the foot upward so toes point toward the ceiling.

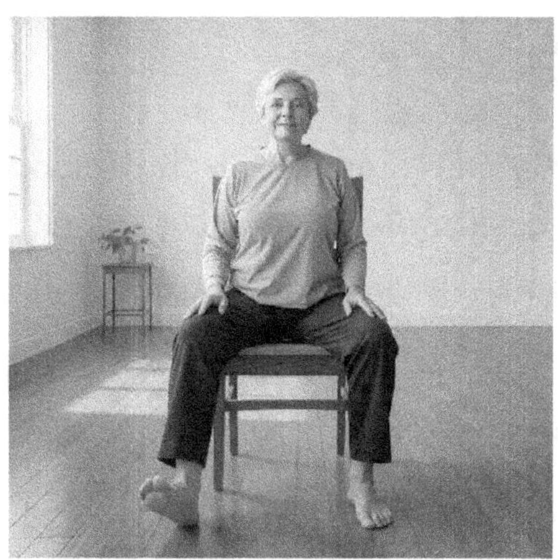

Step 3: Hold and Breathe

At the extended position, pause for one breath cycle. Notice the mild engagement along the top of the thigh. Keep the torso upright and the shoulders relaxed.

Step 4: Return on the Exhale

On the exhale, slowly lower the foot back to the floor and slide it back to starting position. Let the exhale guide the return.

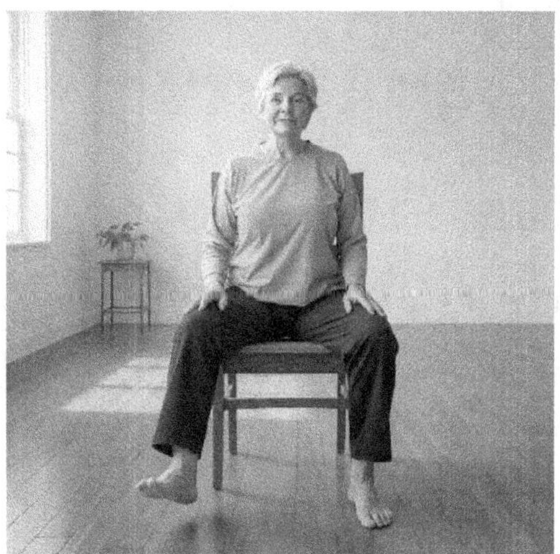

Repetitions: Three to five full cycles alternating sides per session.

Modification: For significant knee stiffness, limit the extension to a very small slide forward. Even a few inches maintains the neuromuscular activation benefit.

3.3.3 Exercise 3: Gentle Side Reaches

Purpose: To stretch the lateral muscles of the torso, improve thoracic spine mobility, open the intercostal muscles for deeper breathing, and cultivate fluid reaching movement.

Starting position: Sit upright, feet flat on the floor hip-width apart, hands resting lightly on the thighs.

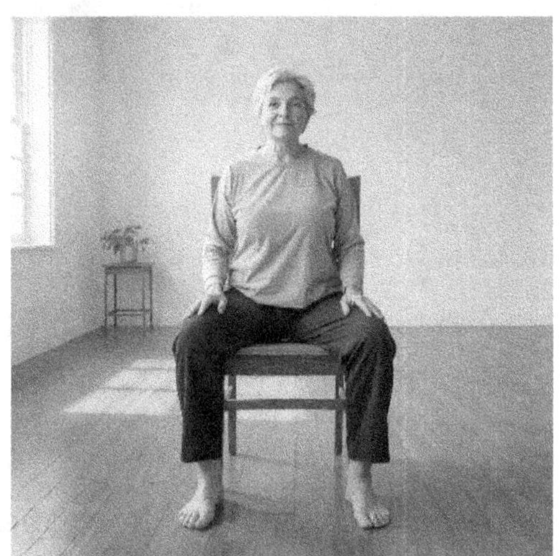

Step 1: Ground and Lengthen

Press both feet gently into the floor. Take one slow breath. On the exhale, feel the crown of the head rise slightly.

Step 2: Float Right Arm on the Inhale

On your inhale, sweep the right arm upward and outward in a wide arc from the thigh, past the side of the body, upward toward the ceiling. The left hand remains on the left thigh for stability.

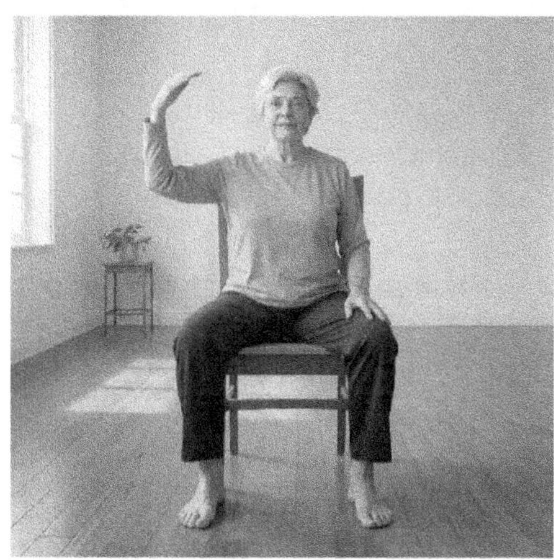

Step 3: Reach and Allow the Incline

At the peak of the inhale with the right arm extended upward, allow the body to incline gently to the left in response to the reach. Feel the long line of stretch from the right hip through the waist, through the ribs, through the arm, and out through the fingertips.

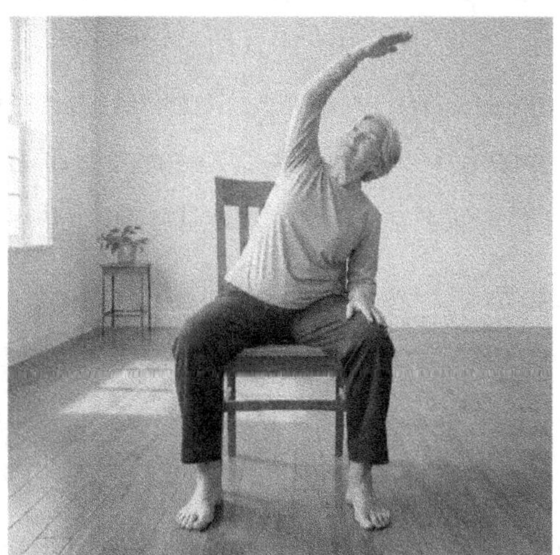

Step 4: Return and Flow

On the exhale, sweep the right arm back down through its arc toward the lap. As it approaches, allow the left arm to begin its upward sweep without a pause, creating a continuous alternating flow.

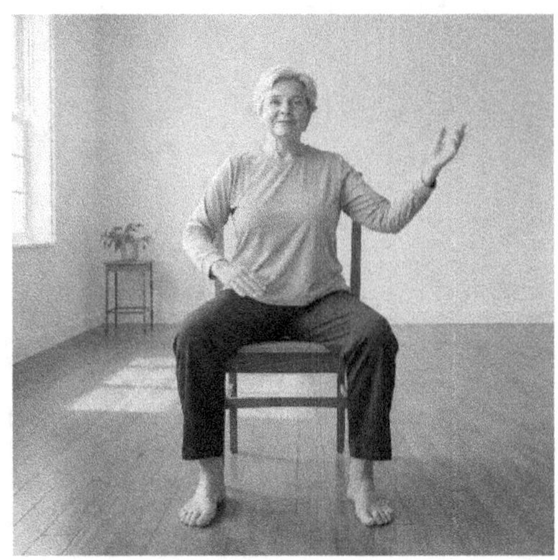

Repetitions: Three to four full cycles alternating sides per session.

Modification: If reaching overhead causes shoulder discomfort, limit the arm sweep to a forward diagonal rather than full overhead, keeping the lateral stretch benefit while reducing the shoulder demand.

Bringing the Three Foundations Together

These three elements, breath, posture, and basic movement, are not three separate things. They are one practice expressed through three lenses. When your breath is coordinated with your movement, your posture naturally improves. When your posture is aligned, your breath deepens. When your movements are slow and intentional, both breath and posture regulate themselves.

In your first practice sessions, attend to each element separately. Over the first week you will begin to notice moments where they come together naturally, where the breath leads a movement without your deliberate management of it, where an arm sweeps through its arc with a quality of ease that surprises you.

Those moments are what this chapter has been preparing you for.

Chapter 4: Common Chair Tai Chi Movements

By now you have spent time with the three pillars of Chair Tai Chi: breath, posture, and the introductory movements that gave you a felt sense of how they work together. Chapter 3 opened the door. This chapter walks you through it.

The movements here are the core vocabulary of your four-week program. Each movement has its own purpose, its own physical benefit, and its own relationship to breath and alignment. Together they form the sequences you will practice daily across the coming weeks.

One important note: the Arm Swings and Side Reaches introduced in Chapter 3 laid the foundation for Sections 4.1 and 4.2. Those sections now build on that foundation with refinements and greater movement detail rather than repeating the basics from scratch.

4.1 Seated Arm Swings

Building on the Foundation

In Chapter 3, you practiced floating the arms forward and upward as a breath-coordination exercise. The Seated Arm Swing expands this into a fuller, more dynamic movement that adds a gentle pendulum quality, directional variation, and conscious engagement of the shoulder girdle.

The shoulder joint has the greatest range of motion of any joint in the body. In sedentary older adults, the muscles and connective tissue surrounding the shoulder commonly tighten and shorten due to prolonged forward-facing postures. Regular, full-arc arm movement is one of the most effective ways to counteract this progressive restriction.

A student in one of my assisted living classes had not been able to reach the back of her own head without pain for nearly three years due to shoulder stiffness. After four weeks of daily Arm Swings, she reported combing her hair without discomfort for the first time since her early seventies. Her physical therapist confirmed measurable improvements in external shoulder rotation at her next appointment.

Starting position: Sit upright, feet flat on the floor hip-width apart. Hands rest loosely in the lap, palms facing inward toward the thighs. Shoulders dropped and relaxed.

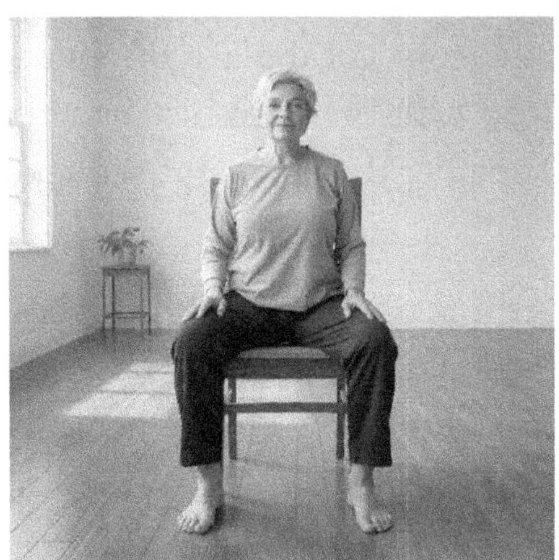

Step 1: Settle and Connect

Take one full breath cycle before beginning. On the exhale, let the shoulders drop fully. Feel the slight heaviness of relaxed hands in the lap.

Step 2: Forward Swing on the Inhale

On your inhale, allow both arms to swing gently forward and upward, elbows soft. Allow a very slight natural momentum rather than a deliberate lift. Rise to shoulder height or whatever is comfortable. Palms face downward as the arms rise.

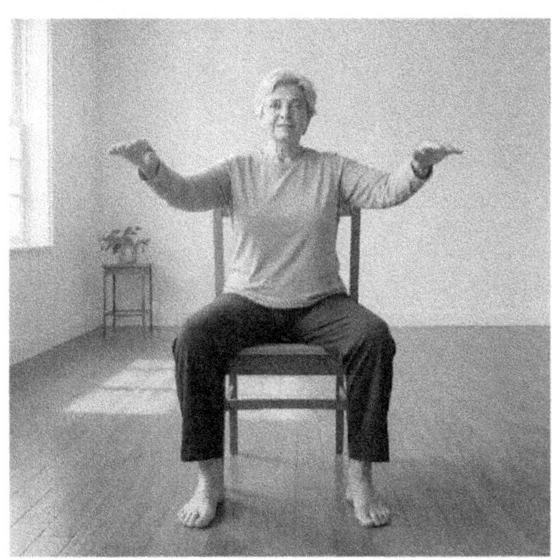

Step 3: Arc Outward at the Peak

At shoulder height, without pausing, allow the arms to gently arc outward, opening slightly away from each other, so that by the time they begin descending they are slightly wider than shoulder-width apart.

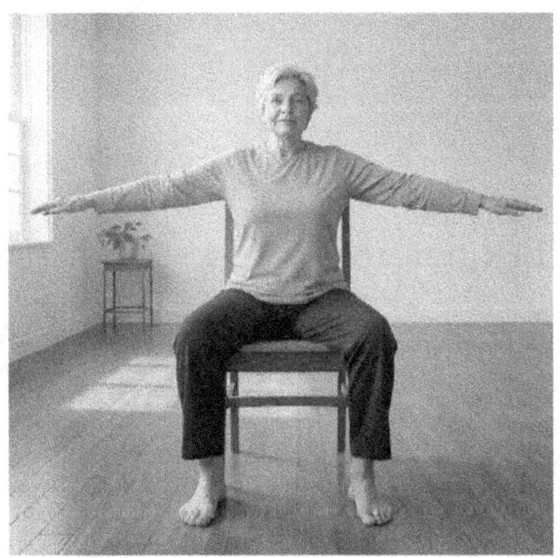

Step 4: Return Swing on the Exhale

As you exhale, allow the arms to swing back downward and slightly inward, returning naturally to the lap guided by the exhale and gravity. Let the hands land softly without any abrupt stopping.

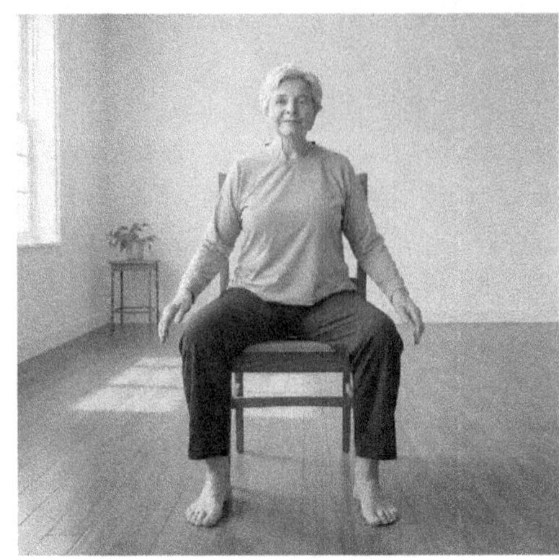

Repetitions: Six to eight full cycles per session.

Modification: Those with shoulder impingement or limited range of motion should keep the arc smaller, rising only to chest height and omitting the outward arc at the peak until range of motion improves.

4.2 Seated Side Reaches

From Introduction to Full Expression

The Side Reach was first introduced in Chapter 3 as a single-arm stretch. Here it develops into a fuller bilateral expression that alternates sides in a flowing sequence and adds greater attention to the spinal rotation that naturally accompanies lateral reaching.

The thoracic spine tends to become progressively stiff in sedentary older adults, restricting breathing depth, contributing to rounded upper back posture, and limiting the quality of all upper body movement. The Seated Side Reach directly and accessibly maintains and restores thoracic mobility.

Starting position: Sit upright, feet flat on the floor hip-width apart. Both hands rest lightly on the thighs. Spine long. Shoulders dropped.

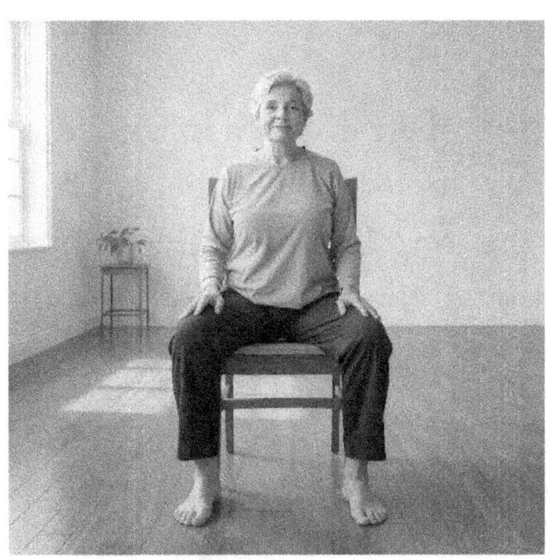

Step 1: Ground and Lengthen

Press both feet firmly into the floor. Take one slow breath. On the exhale, feel the crown of the head rise slightly as the spine gently draws upward.

Step 2: Float Right Arm on the Inhale

On your inhale, sweep the right arm upward and outward in a wide, generous arc from the thigh, past the side of the body and upward toward the ceiling. The left hand remains on the left thigh. As the right arm rises, allow the right side of the torso to naturally lengthen.

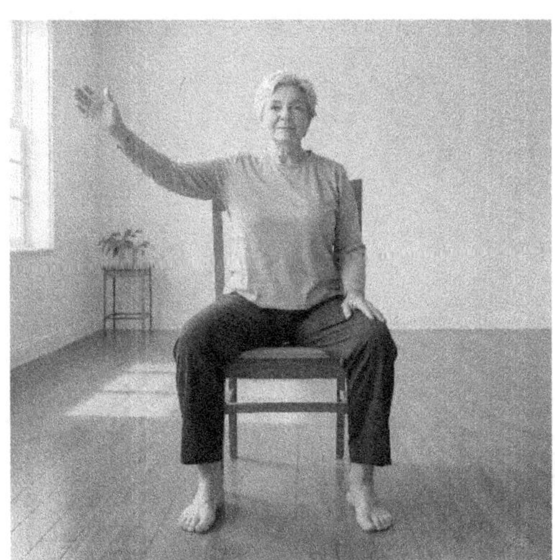

Step 3: Reach and Allow the Incline

At the peak of the inhale with the right arm extended upward, allow the body to incline gently to the left in response to the reach. The left sit bone presses more firmly into the seat. Feel the long line of stretch from the right hip through the waist, through the ribs, through the arm, and out through the fingertips.

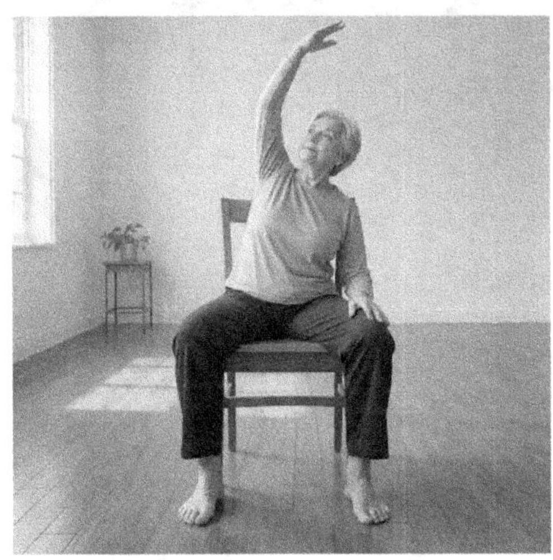

Step 4: Return and Flow to the Left

On the exhale, sweep the right arm back down through its arc toward the lap. As it approaches, allow the left arm to begin its upward sweep without a pause, creating a flowing, alternating rhythm like the gentle rhythm of a slow wave.

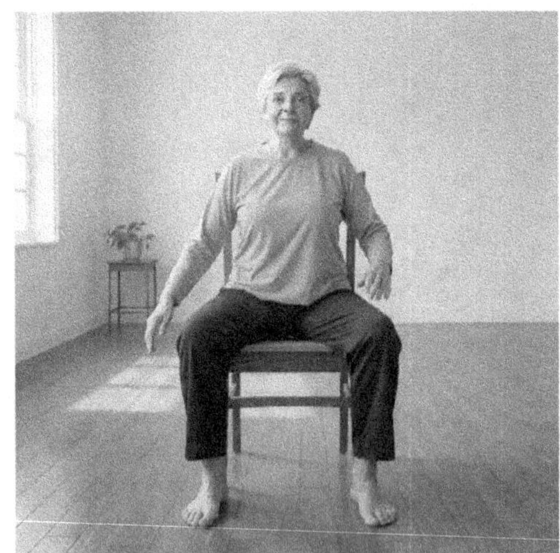

Repetitions: Four to six full cycles alternating sides per session.

Modification: Those with shoulder limitations can perform the reach with the elbow bent, sweeping the hand up to ear level rather than full overhead extension.

4.3 Seated Knee Lifts

A New Movement: Lower Body Activation

Where the Arm Swings and Side Reaches work primarily through the upper body and torso, the Seated Knee Lift introduces deliberate lower body activation. It builds on the Leg Extension from Chapter 3 by changing the primary action from extending the leg outward to lifting the knee upward, which engages a different set of muscles and produces complementary benefits.

The hip flexors and quadriceps engaged here are the muscles most directly responsible for stepping, climbing stairs, and rising from a chair, making them among the most functionally important muscle groups for daily independence in older adults.

Starting position: Sit upright, slightly forward on the seat. Hands rest lightly on the armrests or thighs. Feet flat on the floor hip-width apart.

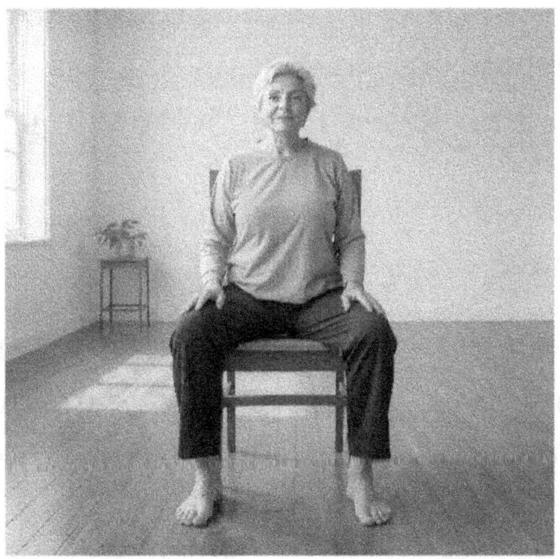

Step 1: Root and Stabilize

Ground both feet into the floor. Take one slow breath cycle. On the exhale, engage the lower abdominals very gently, drawing the navel slightly inward without holding the breath.

Step 2: Lift the Right Knee on the Inhale

On your inhale, slowly lift the right foot off the floor by raising the right knee upward. The foot naturally follows the knee. Aim to lift the knee to a comfortable height. The left foot remains firmly grounded.

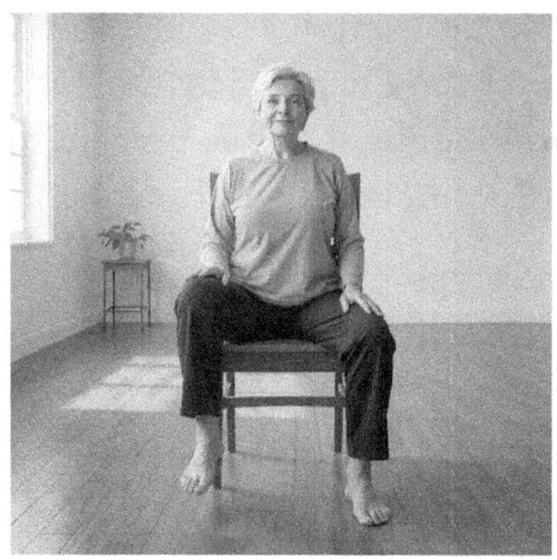

Step 3: Hold at the Peak

At the peak of the inhale, hold the knee at its lifted height for one natural breath pause. Keep the torso upright. Resist the tendency to lean backward as the knee rises.

Step 4: Lower on the Exhale

On the exhale, slowly lower the right foot back to the floor, placing it down with control rather than letting it drop. Feel the foot making deliberate, grounded contact with the floor before shifting attention to the left side.

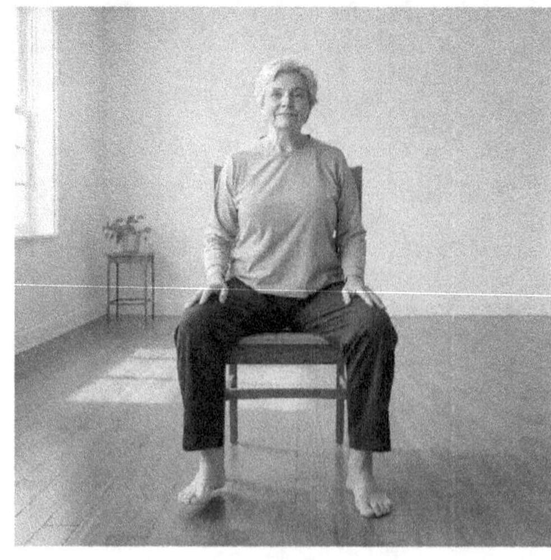

Repetitions: Four to six full cycles alternating sides per session.

Variation: After lifting the knee, add a gentle leg extension from the knee, straightening the lower leg slightly before returning the foot to the floor.

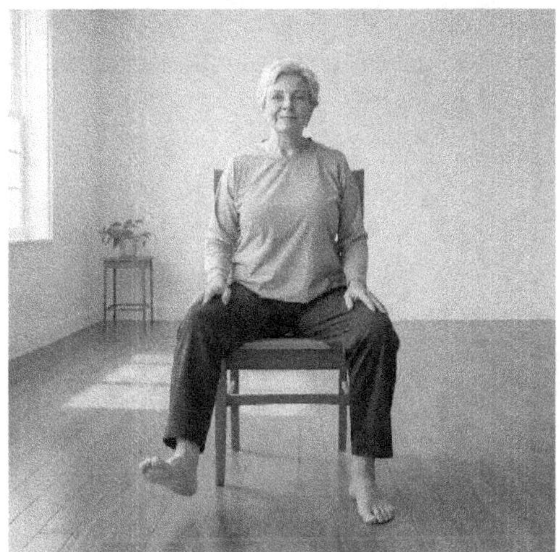

Modification: For hip replacements or significant hip arthritis, simply raise the heel off the floor with minimal knee elevation.

4.4 Tai Chi Push Movements

The Language of Tai Chi in Motion

The Push movement draws directly from one of the fundamental gestures of traditional Tai Chi form, known in Chinese as "An," meaning pressing or pushing forward. In Chair Tai Chi it is adapted as a forward and slightly downward bilateral push from the chest, executed with the full weight of slow breath and deliberate intention.

Unlike the arm-swinging movements that rely on pendulum momentum, the Push is entirely internally driven. It requires the full cooperation of breath, posture, and attention. The muscles engaged are the same ones used in pushing open a heavy door, steadying oneself against a surface, and any activity requiring controlled forward force.

Starting position: Sit upright, feet flat on the floor. Bring both hands to chest level, palms facing forward and slightly downward, fingers pointing upward. Elbows bent and positioned in front of the ribcage just below shoulder level.

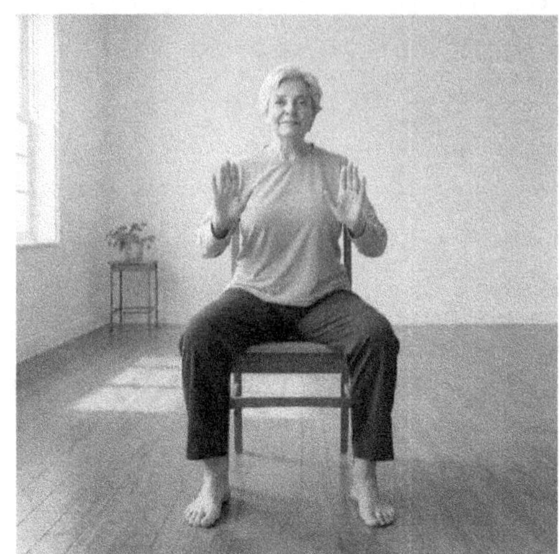

Step 1: Gather and Root

Feel the weight of the hands at chest level. Ground the feet firmly. Take one slow breath to settle and find the posture. Notice the gentle engagement of the shoulder muscles holding the hands at chest height without strain.

Step 2: Begin the Push on the Exhale

As you begin a long, slow exhale, press both palms forward and very slightly downward, as though pressing against a resistant but yielding surface at chest level. The arms extend slowly and steadily as the exhale progresses.

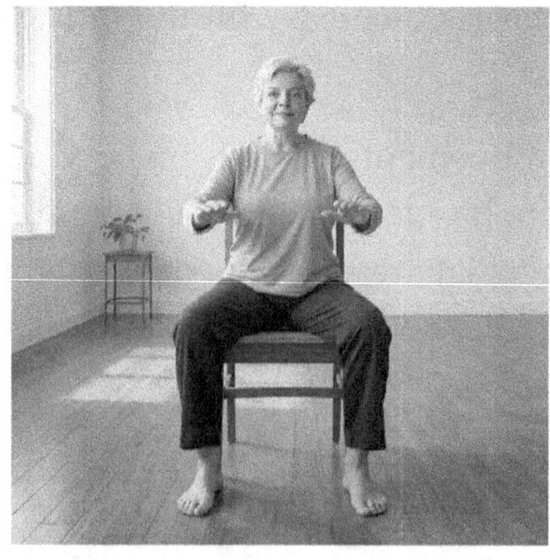

Step 3: Full Extension at the End of the Exhale

By the time the exhale completes, the arms are extended forward with elbows remaining softly bent, palms facing forward, fingers pointing upward. Do not lock the elbows. Pause briefly at the full extension.

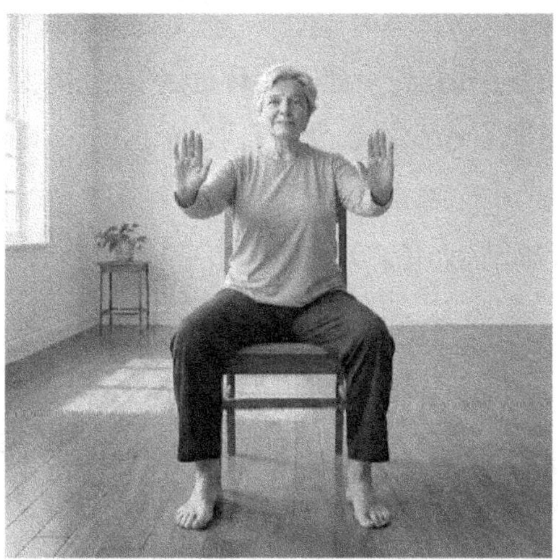

Step 4: Return on the Inhale

As you inhale, draw both hands back slowly toward the chest, bending the elbows and returning through the path of the push. The wrists lead the return, drawing inward as though gathering something toward the center of the chest.

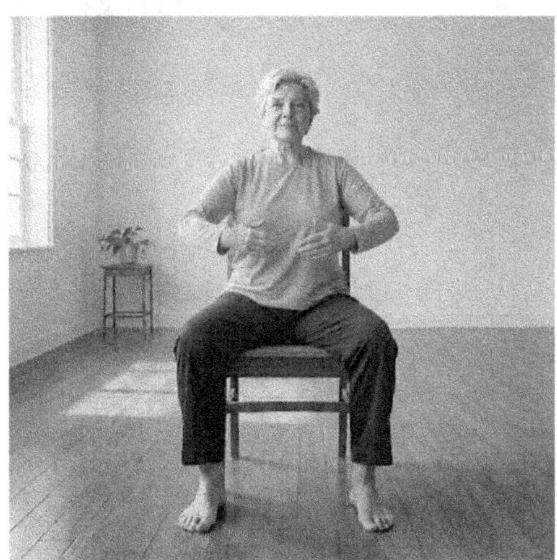

Repetitions: Four to six full push-and-return cycles per session.

Modification: Those with shoulder limitations can perform a smaller push, extending the arms only partially forward while maintaining the same breath coordination and intentional quality.

4.5 Seated Tai Chi Walks

Walking Without Standing

The Seated Tai Chi Walk simulates the alternating leg and arm coordination of walking, performed entirely from the chair. It engages the hip flexors, quadriceps, and core stabilizers while training the cross-body neural coordination fundamental to smooth, confident gait in daily life.

For many seniors, the connection between the right arm and left leg, and between the left arm and right leg, has become less synchronized over years of reduced activity. The Seated Tai Chi Walk directly trains these pathways in a safe, seated environment where the benefits then transfer to actual walking.

Starting position: Sit upright with feet flat on the floor hip-width apart. Arms hang loosely at the sides, hands level with the hips. Spine long, shoulders dropped.

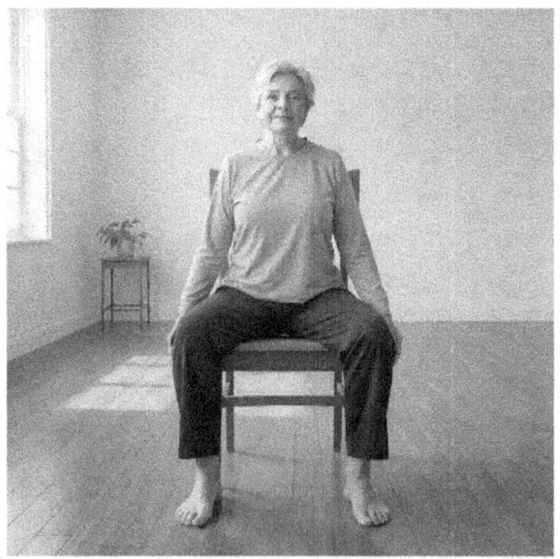

Step 1: Find the Rhythm of the Breath

Before beginning any limb movement, breathe for two full cycles and feel the natural rhythm of the breath. The Seated Tai Chi Walk uses a longer breath cycle, inhaling across two steps and exhaling across two steps, so breathing feels unhurried even as the leg and arm movements alternate continuously.

Step 2: Lift Right Knee and Swing Left Arm

On the first count of your inhale, lift the right knee upward while simultaneously allowing the left arm to swing forward from the hip, as though taking a natural walking step. The right arm moves slightly backward, mirroring the opposite-arm-opposite-leg coordination of real walking.

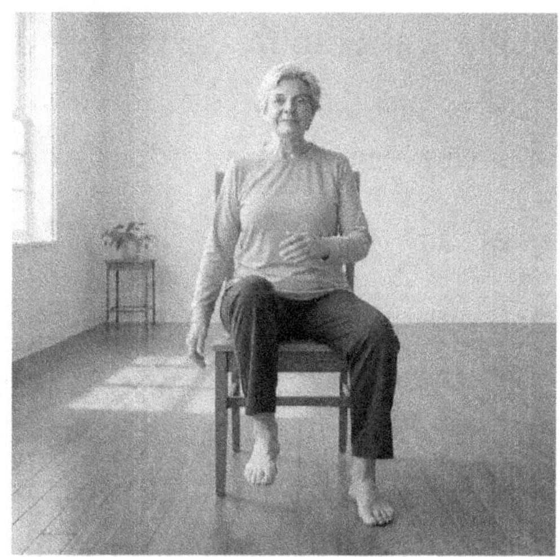

Step 3: Transition to Left Knee and Right Arm

On the second count of the inhale, lower the right foot back to the floor while lifting the left knee upward, simultaneously swinging the right arm forward while the left arm moves slightly back. The transition is smooth and continuous, no pause between sides.

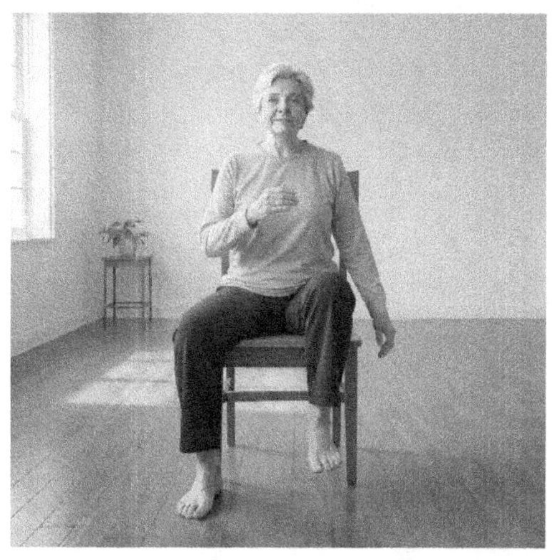

Step 4: Continue Through the Exhale

On the exhale, continue the alternating pattern for two more counts, right and left. Allow the rhythm to find its own natural pace, one that matches your breath without requiring counting. The arms and legs should begin to feel like a coordinated whole.

Repetitions: Six to eight full breath cycles, approximately eight to twelve alternating steps per side, per session.

Modification: Those with significant hip flexor tightness can simply raise the heel off the floor while pressing the toes down, combined with the arm swing. Cross-body coordination training is preserved even at this minimal range.

Putting the Movements Together

The five movements in this chapter now give you a complete, balanced practice session when combined with the breath and posture foundations of Chapter 3. The Arm Swings warm the shoulder girdle. The Side Reaches open the thoracic spine and lateral body. The Knee Lifts activate the hip flexors and lower body. The Push builds coordinated upper body strength and intentional force. The Seated Tai Chi Walk synthesizes everything into the most functionally relevant movement pattern of daily life.

Practiced in this order, each movement prepares the body for the next. Learn them well now. The time you invest here will pay dividends for every session that follows.

Chapter 5: Week 1 — Gentle Introduction to Movements

Welcome to your first week of practice. This is where everything you have read becomes something you actually feel.

Your only job this week is to show up. Don't worry about getting the moves perfect or feeling a 'burn.' Just get used to sitting in the chair, taking a breath, and moving your body with intention. If you feel a little awkward at first, you're doing it right.

Each daily session this week follows the same simple structure: a warm-up to prepare the joints, a breath and posture check-in to anchor your attention, and the introductory movements that form the foundation of your practice. Keep the same chair, the same space, and the same general time of day whenever possible. Show up. Move gently. Breathe. That is the entire assignment for Week 1.

5.1 Warm-Up: Gentle Stretches

Why Warming Up Matters

Cold joints and tight muscles do not move well, and asking them to move through Tai Chi sequences without preparation is the most common cause of the minor discomforts that discourage beginners from continuing. The warm-up is not optional. It is the first movement of your practice.

The three warm-up exercises below take approximately two to three minutes and systematically prepare the joints most involved in Chair Tai Chi: the neck, the shoulders, and the wrists.

5.1.1 Warm-Up Exercise 1: Neck Rolls

Purpose: To release habitual tension in the cervical spine and surrounding neck muscles, improving the range of cervical motion and reducing the stiffness many people carry from sleeping positions or prolonged screen time.

Starting position: Sit upright, feet flat, hands in lap. Spine long, shoulders dropped.

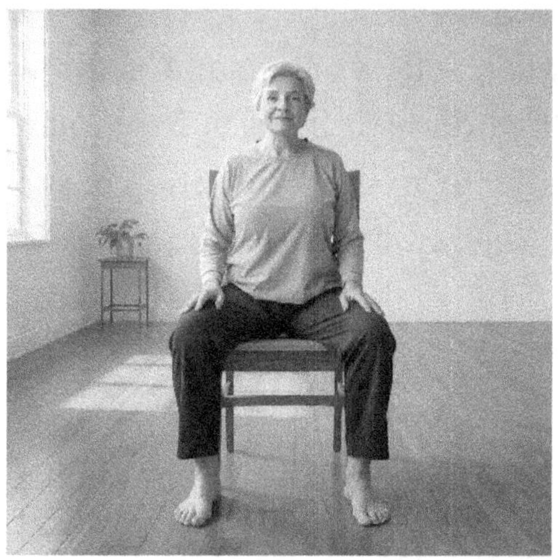

Step 1: Take one full breath. On the exhale, let the chin drop gently toward the chest and feel the stretch through the back of the neck.

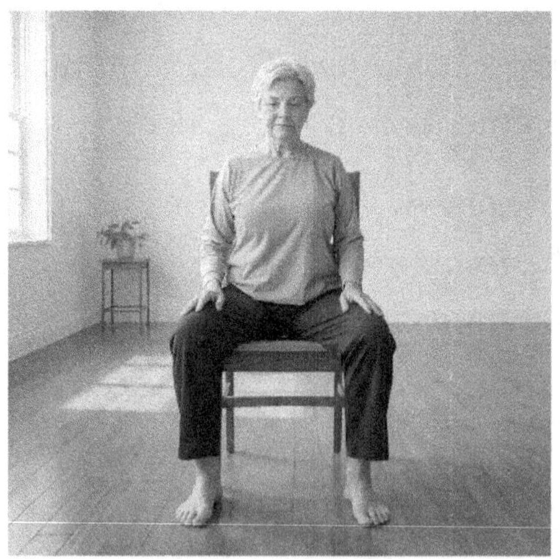

Step 2: Inhaling, slowly roll the head to the right, bringing the right ear toward the right shoulder. Keep the shoulder down; bring the ear to the shoulder, not the shoulder to the ear.

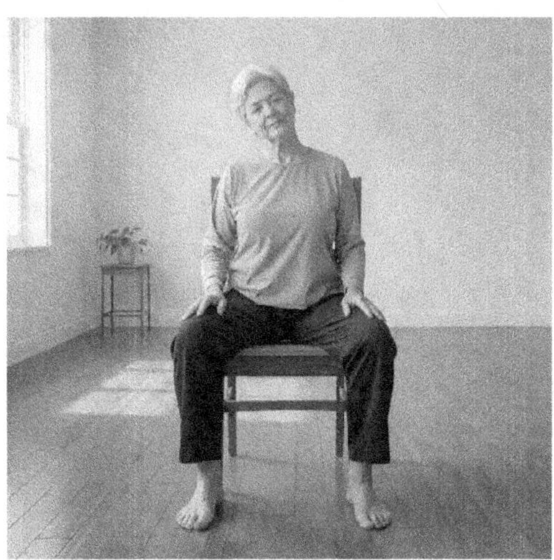

Step 3: Take a natural breath pause at the right side, then exhale as you roll the chin slowly back down toward the chest through the front arc.

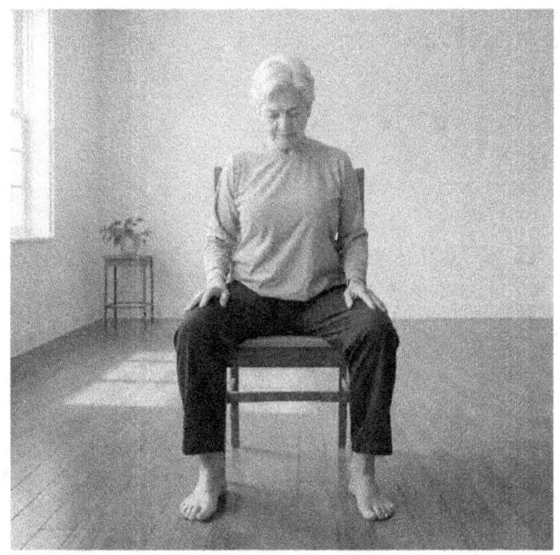

Step 4: Inhaling, continue rolling to the left, left ear moving toward the left shoulder. Pause, breathe, then exhale and return the chin to center and slowly raise the head to neutral.

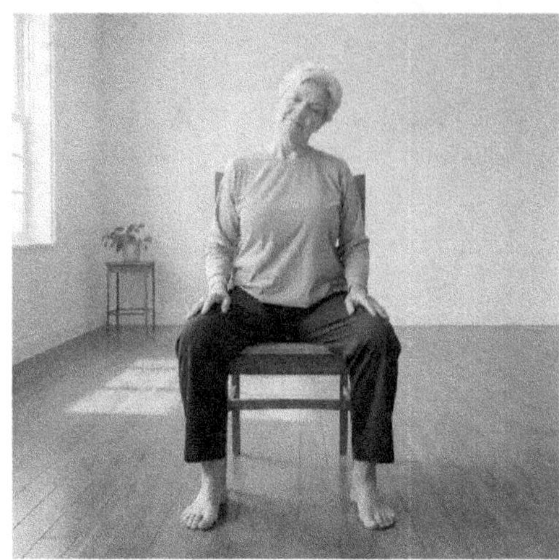

Repetitions: Two full slow rolls in each direction.

Important note: Do not roll the head backward to complete a full circle. Keep all neck movement in the forward half-arc only.

5.1.2 Warm-Up Exercise 2: Shoulder Rolls

Purpose: To warm the shoulder joint, release upper trapezius tension, and activate circulation through the shoulder girdle before the arm movements of the main practice.

Starting position: Sit upright, feet flat, hands resting loosely in the lap. Shoulders dropped.

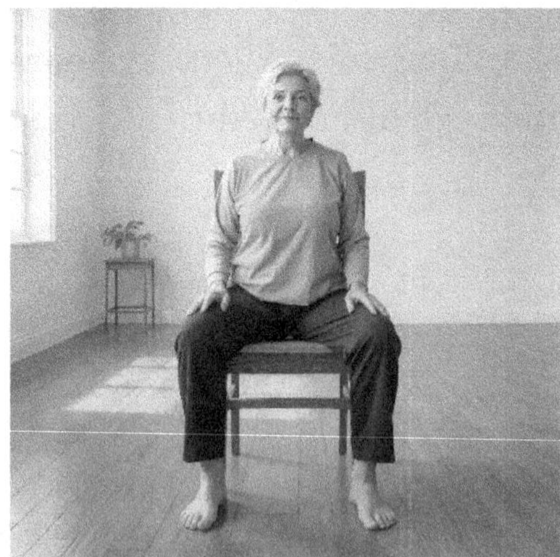

Step 1: Inhale and draw both shoulders upward toward the ears in a slow, deliberate shrug.

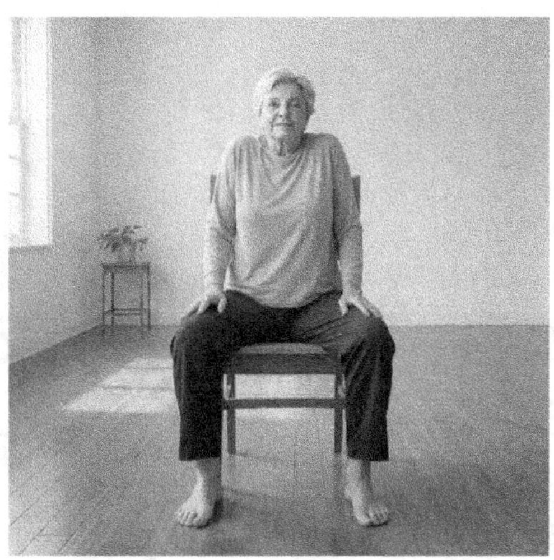

Step 2: At the top of the inhale, roll both shoulders back, squeezing the shoulder blades gently toward each other. Then exhale as the shoulders roll downward, releasing completely away from the ears.

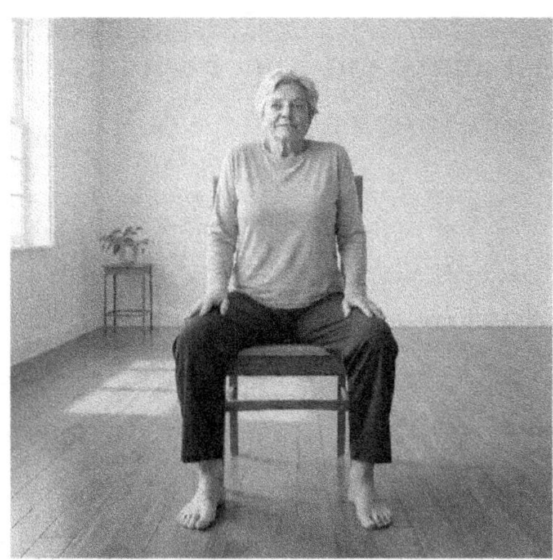

Step 3: Continue the roll forward in a smooth circle, returning to the starting position. After three forward circles, reverse direction for three circles.

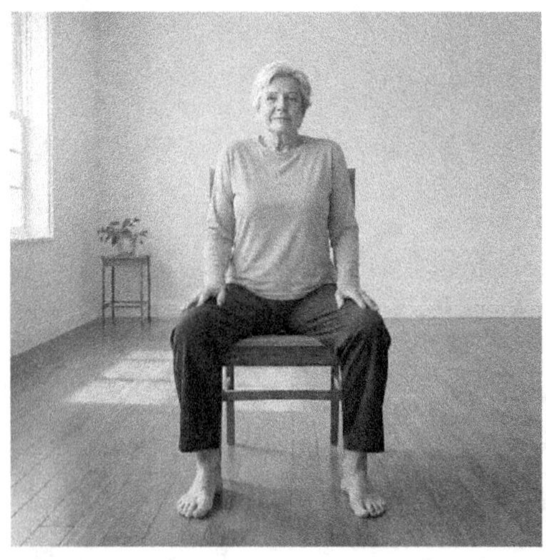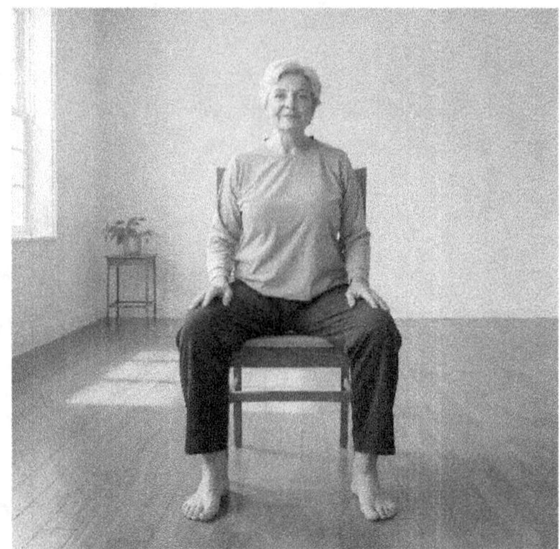

Repetitions: Three circles forward, three circles backward.

5.1.3 Warm-Up Exercise 3: Wrist Flexions and Circles

Purpose: To warm the wrist joints and finger tendons, improving circulation and mobility in the hands before movements requiring arm extension and push gestures.

Starting position: Sit upright. Raise both forearms to lap level, elbows gently bent at the sides, palms facing downward.

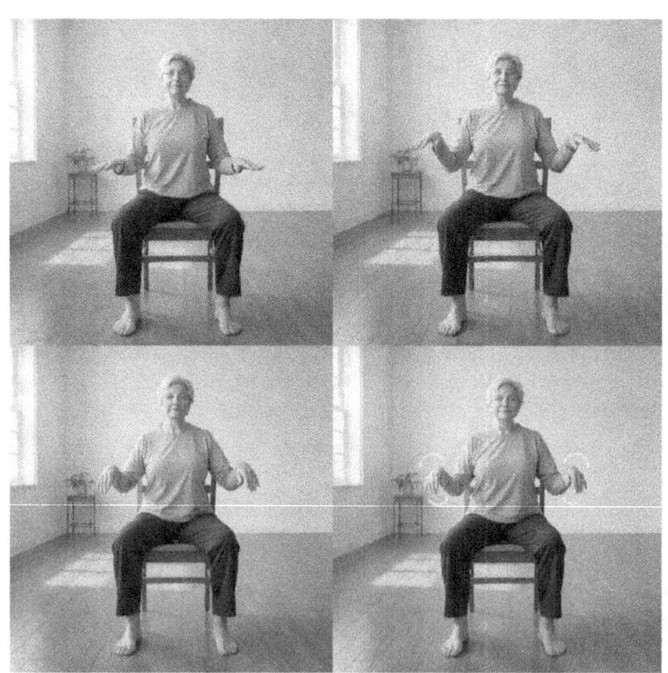

Step 1: Slowly flex both wrists downward, fingertips pointing toward the floor. Hold for one breath.

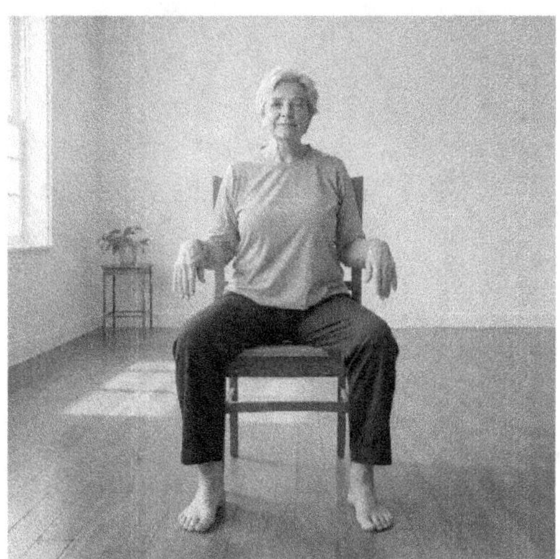

Step 2: Slowly extend both wrists upward, fingertips pointing toward the ceiling. Hold for one breath.

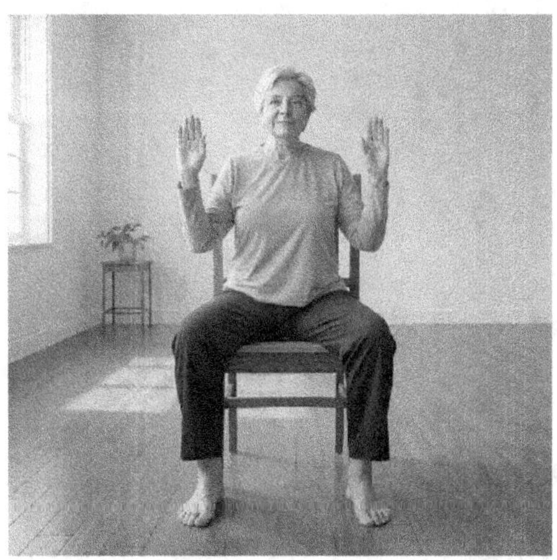

Step 3: Make loose, relaxed fists.

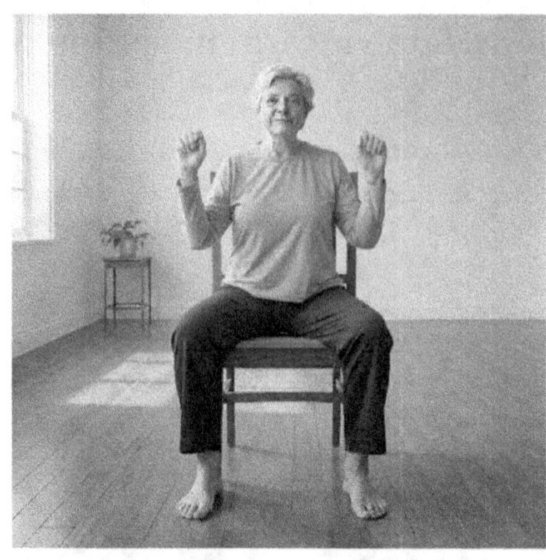

Step 4: Begin slow wrist circles in one direction for four circles. After completing four circles

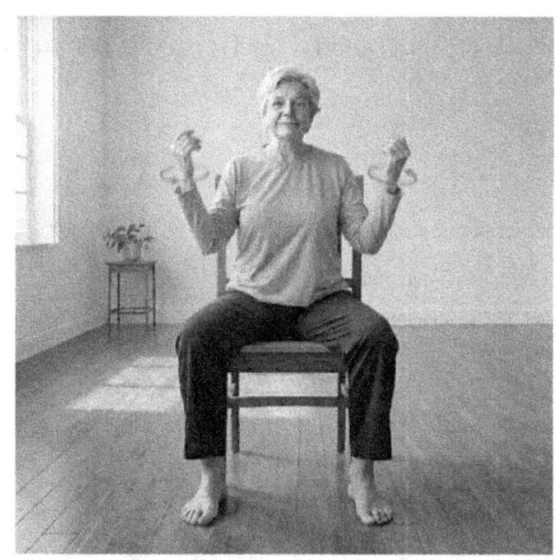

Step 5: Reverse the direction of the wrist then circle for four circles.

Step 6: Finish by spreading all fingers wide, holding for two breaths, then releasing.

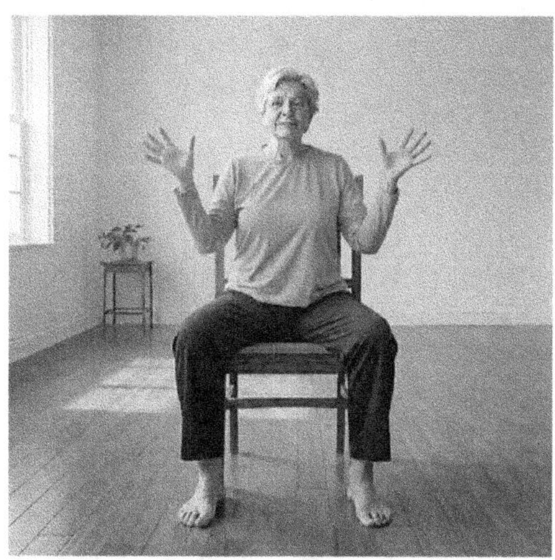

Repetitions: One full sequence as described.

5.2 Basic Breathing and Posture

Your Daily Check-In

After the warm-up, take sixty seconds for a deliberate breath and posture check-in before beginning any of the movement sequences described in chapter 3. This transition moment is an active recalibration that sets the quality of everything that follows.

By Week 1 you have already read the detailed instruction for both diaphragmatic breathing and seated alignment in Chapter 3. What follows is the condensed, practical version for use at the start of every session throughout the four-week program.

The Week 1 Breath and Posture Check-In

Step 1: Press both feet firmly and evenly into the floor. Feel the ground.

Step 2: Roll the pelvis slightly forward until you feel both sit bones in clear, even contact with the seat.

Step 3: Imagine the thread at the crown of the head drawing gently upward. Let the spine lengthen without stiffening.

Step 4: Take a full breath in, then exhale and let the shoulders drop completely away from the ears.

Step 5: Let the hands rest loosely in the lap, fingers uncurled and soft.

Step 6: Take three full diaphragmatic breaths, belly rising on the inhale and softening on the exhale. Make each exhale slightly longer than each inhale.

By the third breath you should feel measurably more settled than when you sat down.

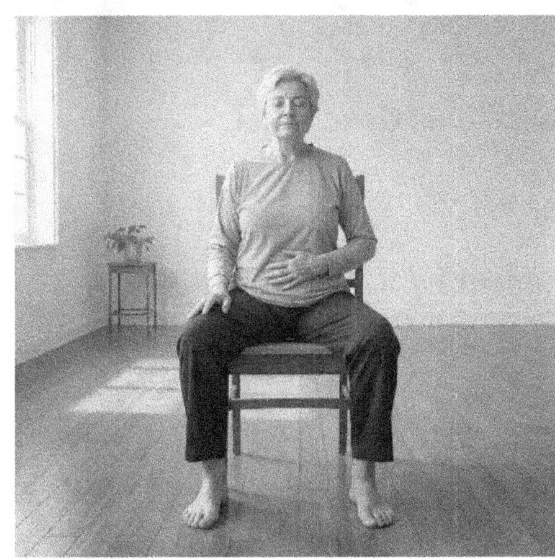

5.3 Seated Forward Bends

A New Movement: Spinal Flexion

The Seated Forward Bend introduces forward flexion, a new direction of spinal movement not yet covered in the program. Where Chapter 3 focused on spinal lengthening and the Side Reaches explored lateral movement, the Seated Forward Bend moves the spine into a gentle, supported forward fold that stretches the entire posterior chain, the muscles running along the back of the body from the base of the skull down through the lumbar spine, gluteals, and hamstrings.

This posterior chain tightness is nearly universal in sedentary older adults. It contributes to lower back pain, postural rounding, and reduced ability to bend forward in daily activities. The Seated Forward Bend addresses it directly without any of the risk that floor-based forward folding would present.

This is a movement of release, not effort. The goal is never to reach a particular depth. The goal is to breathe into the stretch and let gravity do the work gradually and gently.

Starting position: Sit upright on the front half of the chair seat, feet flat on the floor hip-width apart or slightly wider. Hands rest on the thighs. Spine lengthened.

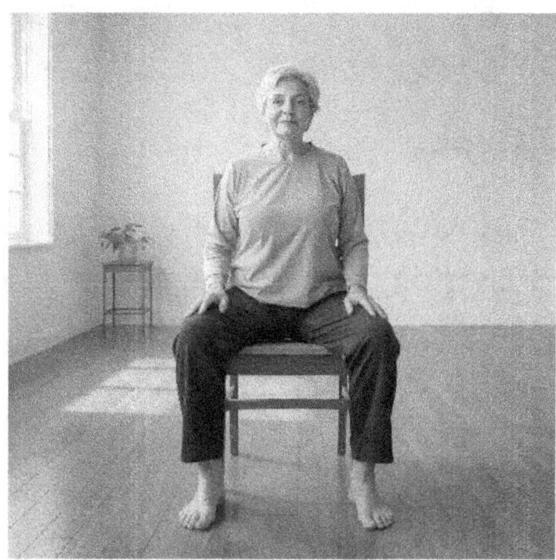

Step 1: Root and Lengthen

Ground the feet. Take a full inhale and feel the spine lengthen upward through the crown of the head.

Step 2: Hinge Forward on the Exhale

On your exhale, hinge the entire torso forward from the hip joint, not the waist. Lead with the chest rather than the head. Allow the hands to slide forward along the thighs toward the knees as the torso lowers.

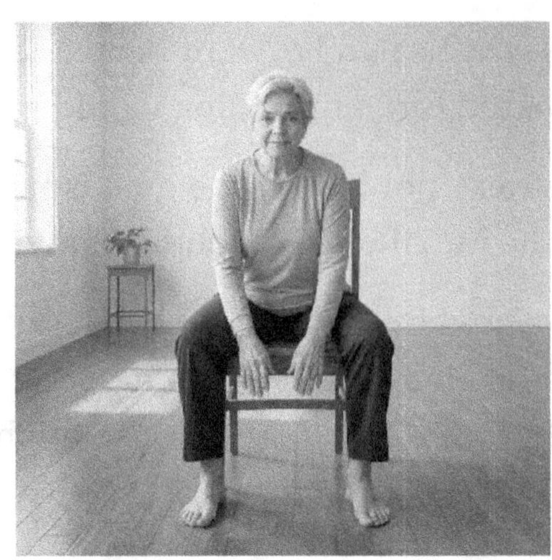

Step 3: Find Your Natural Depth

Lower only as far as is comfortable. For many people in Week 1 this will be a moderate forward lean with hands resting on the knees. The right depth is the one at which you feel a clear but comfortable stretch through the lower back and hamstrings without any strain or gripping.

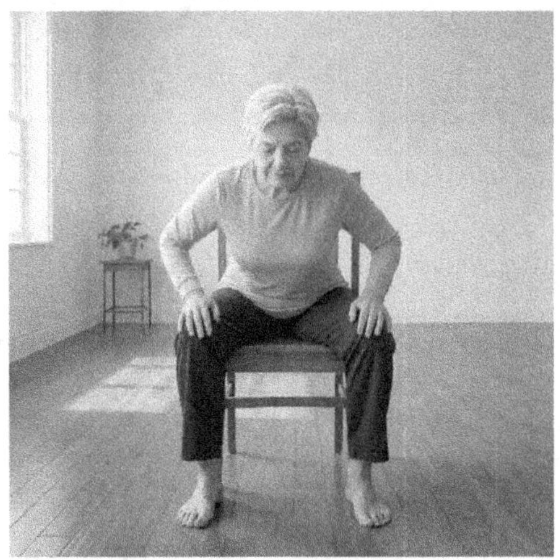

Step 4: Breathe into the Stretch

Hold the forward position for two to three breath cycles. With each exhale, allow the body to release a small amount further forward without forcing. Let gravity and the breath deepen the stretch naturally.

Step 5: Return on an Inhale

On an inhale, press the hands gently into the thighs for support and slowly roll the spine back up to upright, vertebra by vertebra from the base of the spine to the crown of the head. The head arrives upright last.

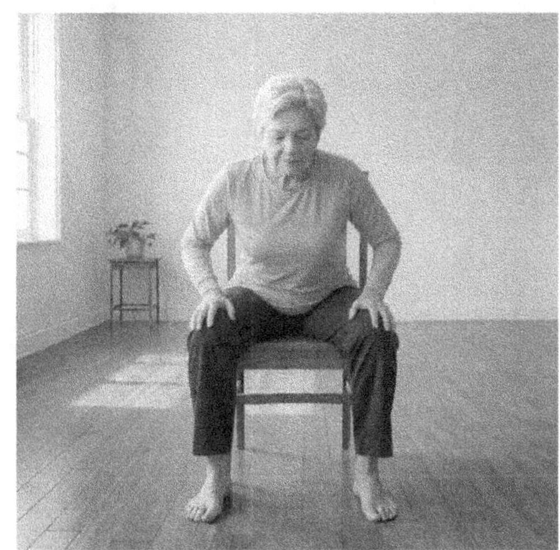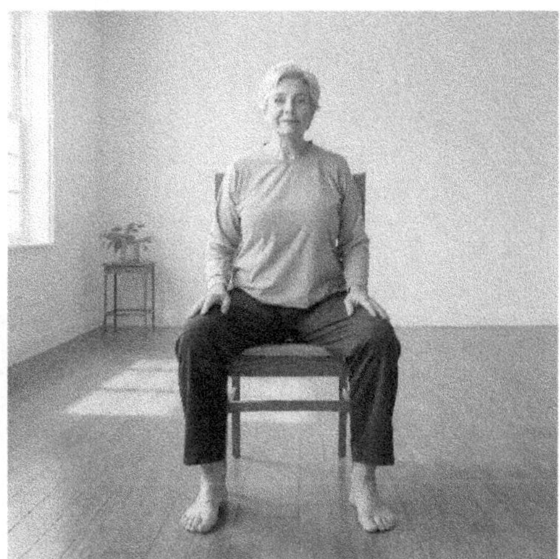

Repetitions: Two to three full cycles per session in Week 1.

Modification: Those with significant lower back conditions or recent spinal surgery should perform only a very minimal forward lean of five to ten degrees from vertical and consult their healthcare provider before deepening the movement.

Closing Week 1: A Note on Consistency Over Intensity

By the end of your first week, you will have practiced the Neck Rolls, Shoulder Rolls, and Wrist Flexions as your daily warm-up. You will have used the Breath and Posture Check-In to anchor each session. And you will have introduced the Seated Forward Bend as the first new movement of your four-week plan.

None of these movements are difficult. That is deliberate. Week 1 is not about challenging your body. It is about building the habit, the daily ten minutes, the consistent space, the reliable chair, the breath-movement connection that makes everything in Weeks 2 through 4 possible. Neuroscience is clear on this: the brain requires consistent repetition to encode new movement patterns. Seven days of gentle, attentive practice does more for your long-term progress than one intense session followed by six days of rest.

You have started something real. Week 2 will build directly on what your body has begun to learn this week.

Chapter 6: Week 2 — Increasing Mobility and Flexibility

You made it through Week 1. That matters more than it might feel like right now.

The first week of any new practice is the hardest, not because the movements are difficult, but because the habit is not yet established. Your body did not yet know what was coming each day. Your mind had not yet learned to look forward to those ten minutes. And yet you showed up, day after day, and moved.

Week 2 builds directly on that foundation. The warm-up routine and breath-posture check-in from Chapter 5 remain your daily anchor. What changes this week is the introduction of four new movement categories that take your practice deeper into spinal rotation, upper body reach, lower body mobility, and lateral balance. Each one is accessible, each one has clear modifications, and each one produces benefits you will begin to feel within the first few sessions.

The word for Week 2 is mobility. Not flexibility in the sense of forcing your body into positions it cannot reach, but the living, functional quality of a body that moves through its available range with ease, without bracing, without hesitation, and without pain. That is what this week cultivates.

6.1 Seated Gentle Twists

Rotation: The Movement Most Often Lost First

Of all the directions the spine can move, rotation is the one most consistently lost in sedentary aging. Flexion and extension, bending forward and backward, are used somewhat in daily life. But full, comfortable spinal rotation, the kind that allows you to turn and look behind you, reach across your body, or twist to speak to someone beside you, tends to decline steadily from middle age onward unless it is specifically and regularly practiced.

The consequences of lost spinal rotation are widespread. It contributes to neck stiffness, because the neck overcompensates for limited thoracic rotation. It reduces the effectiveness of core stabilization, because the oblique muscles that produce rotation also stabilize the spine. It affects gait quality, because healthy walking involves a natural counter-rotation between the upper and lower body. And it affects something harder to quantify but very real: the sense of freedom and ease in the body that comes from being able to turn and reach without limitation.

The Seated Gentle Twist restores this movement safely, from a supported, grounded seat that eliminates any risk of loss of balance and allows the rotation to develop without compensatory movement in the hips or lower back.

Starting position: Sit upright on the front half of the chair seat. Feet flat on the floor, hip-width apart. Hands rest on the thighs. Spine lengthened.

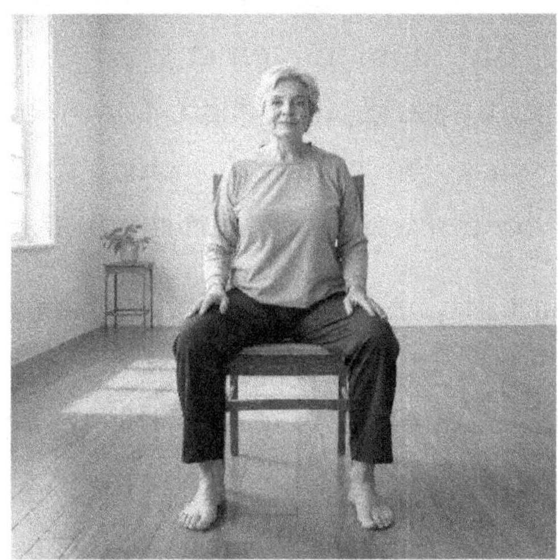

Step 1: Root and Lengthen

Ground both feet firmly. Take one full breath. On the exhale, feel the crown of the head draw upward, lengthening the spine before any rotation begins. This lengthening is essential: rotating a compressed spine produces less range and more risk than rotating a lengthened one.

Step 2: Place the Hands

Bring the right hand to rest on the outside of the left knee. Bring the left hand to rest on the back of the chair seat or the left armrest behind the left hip. These hand positions create the leverage for the rotation without requiring muscular force.

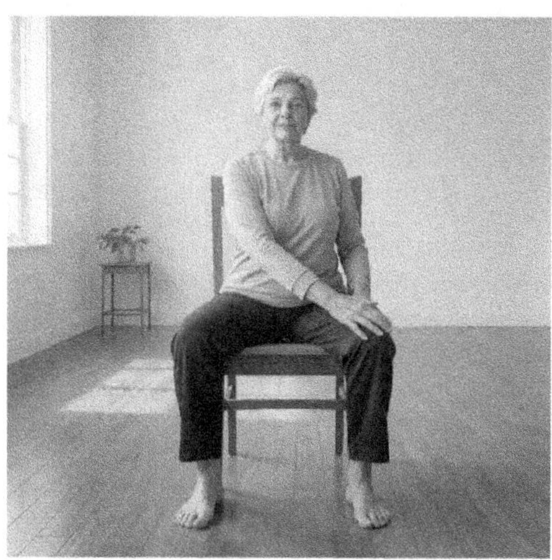

Step 3: Inhale and Lengthen Again

Take a full inhale without beginning the rotation. Use this breath to lengthen the spine once more, as though adding one final inch of hcight before the twist.

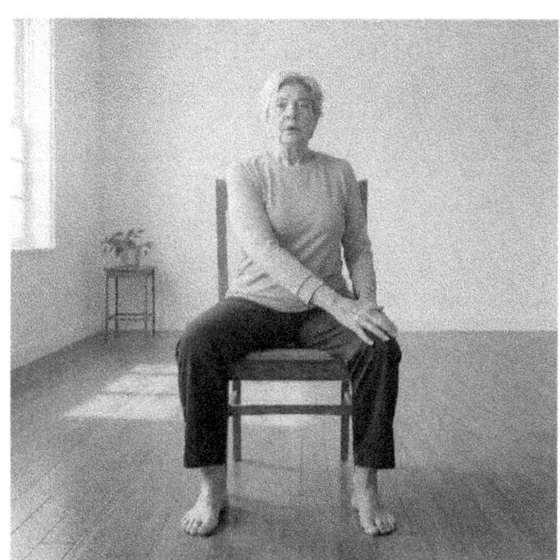

This pre-rotation lengthening is a hallmark of Tai Chi movement and produces measurably greater range than rotating without it.

Step 4: Rotate on the Exhale

As you exhale, slowly rotate the entire upper body to the left, leading with the chest rather than the head. The right hand gently presses into the left knee to deepen the rotation softly. The gaze follows the chest, turning to look over the left shoulder. Rotate only as far as is comfortable, never forcing through resistance.

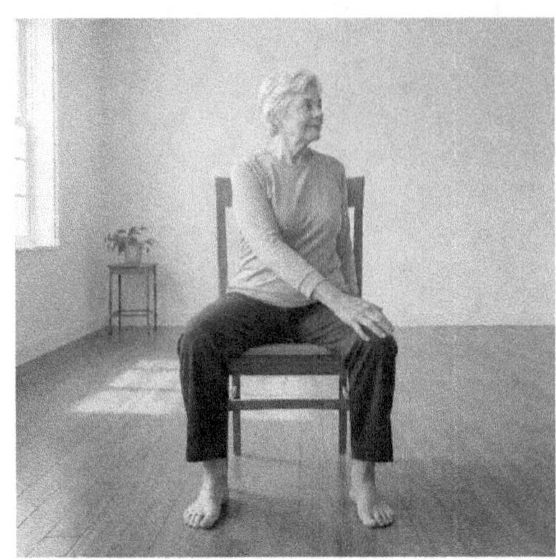

Step 5: Hold and Breathe

Hold the rotated position for two to three breath cycles. With each inhale, lengthen the spine slightly.

With each exhale, allow the rotation to deepen by a small, natural increment without forcing.

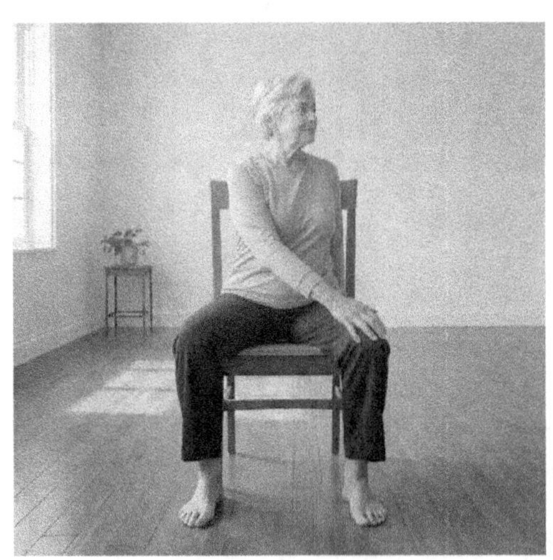

Then inhale.

Gently unwind back to center

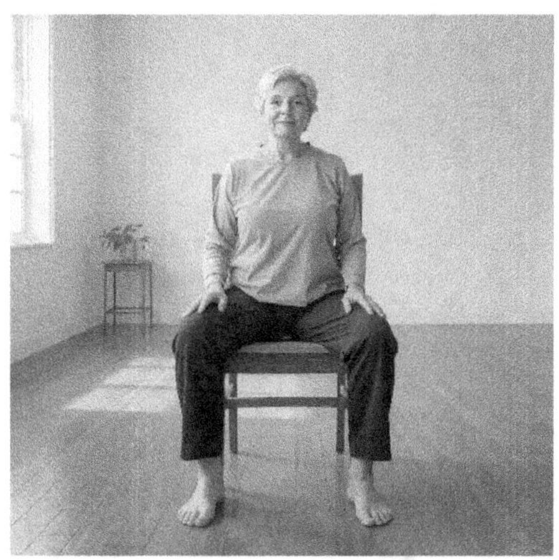

And repeat on the right side.

Repetitions: Two full twists in each direction per session.

Beginner variation: Perform the twist with both hands resting on the thighs, using only the muscles of the core to produce the rotation without any leverage from the hands. This smaller range is fully appropriate for Week 2.

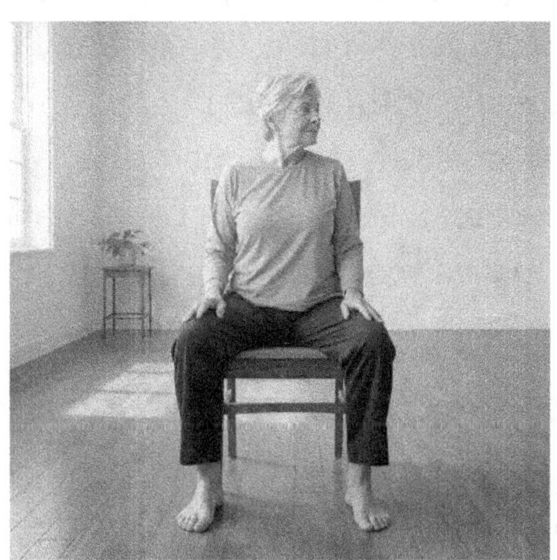

Advanced variation: Extend the outer arm, raising the right arm and pointing it in the direction of the twist as you rotate left, creating a longer rotational line through the body.

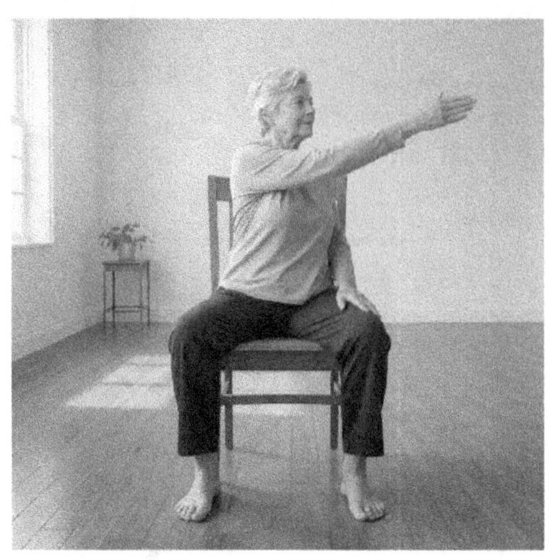

6.2 Breath and Reach Exercises

Upper Body Opening with Intentional Breath

The Breath and Reach exercise builds directly on the Arm Swings and Side Reaches from Chapters 3 and 4, introducing a new dimension: the deliberate combination of a full diaphragmatic breath with a reaching movement that opens the chest, shoulders, and intercostal muscles simultaneously. Where the earlier exercises focused on establishing the breath-movement coordination, the Breath and Reach now uses that coordination as a tool to actively deepen the opening of the upper body with each repetition.

This exercise is particularly effective for seniors who carry chronic tightness through the chest and anterior shoulders, a pattern extremely common in those who have spent years in forward-facing seated postures. Over successive sessions, the combination of expanding breath and reaching arm creates a progressive, gentle stretch through the pectoral muscles and the front of the shoulder that no passive stretching alone can produce.

Starting position: Sit upright, feet flat on the floor hip-width apart. Both arms resting at the sides, hands at hip level. Spine lengthened.

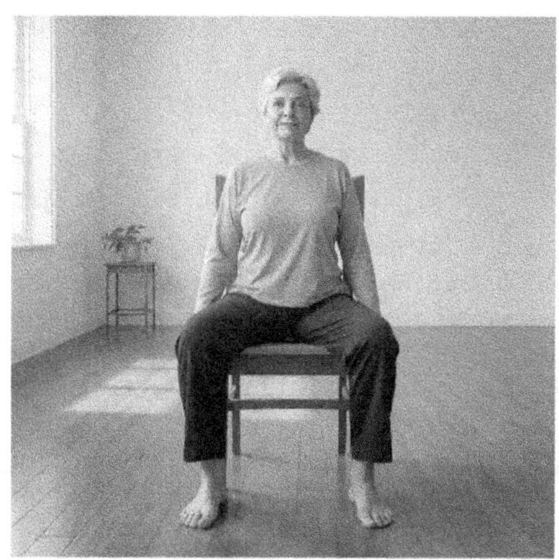

Step 1: Begin at Rest

Settle into the starting position. Take one full breath cycle and let the arms hang completely relaxed at the sides. Feel the weight of the hands and the looseness of the shoulders.

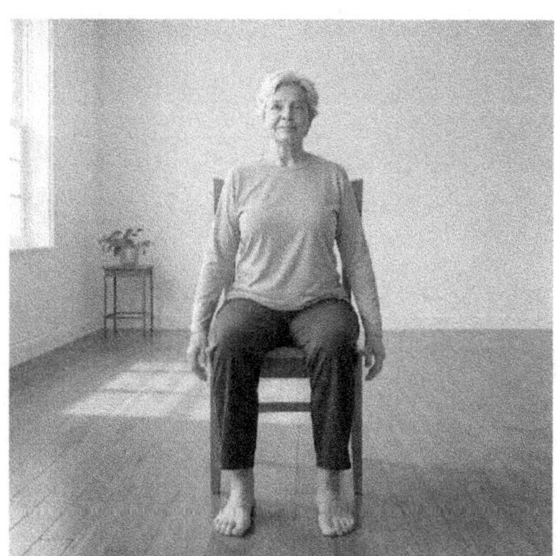

Step 2: Inhale and Sweep Both Arms Wide

On a full, deep inhale, sweep both arms outward and upward in a wide, expansive arc, like wings opening. Allow the chest to open and lift as the arms rise. The movement is generous and unhurried, matching the full length of the inhale. Arms rise to shoulder height or slightly above.

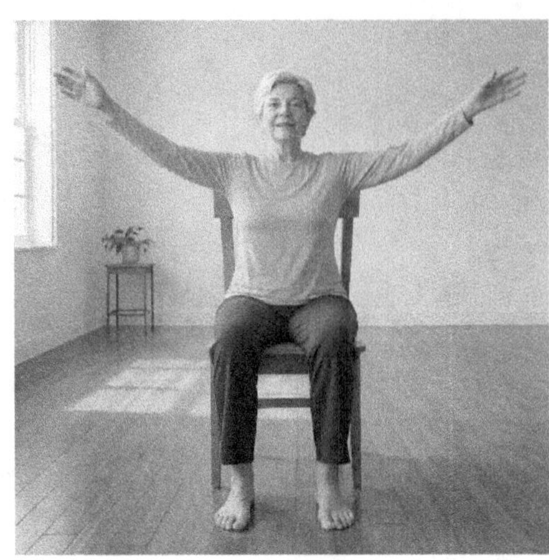

Step 3: Reach at the Peak

At the top of the inhale with arms extended at shoulder height or above, add a gentle additional reach through the fingertips, as though trying to extend the arms one inch further than they have already reached. This reach engages the serratus anterior muscle along the sides of the ribcage and deepens the chest opening further.

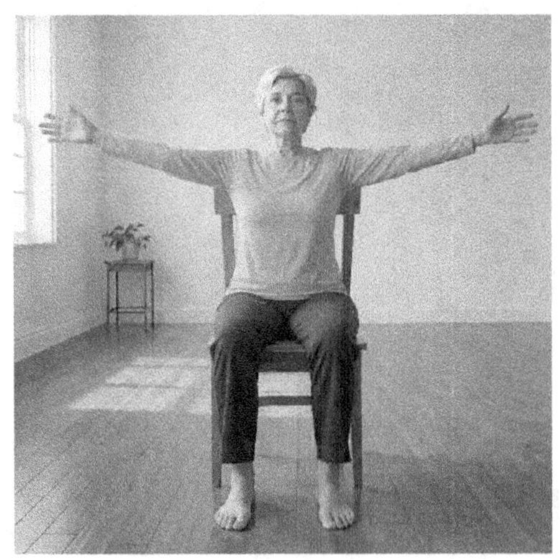

Step 4: Exhale and Draw the Arms Inward

On the exhale, slowly draw both arms inward and downward, crossing them gently across the chest in a self-embracing gesture.

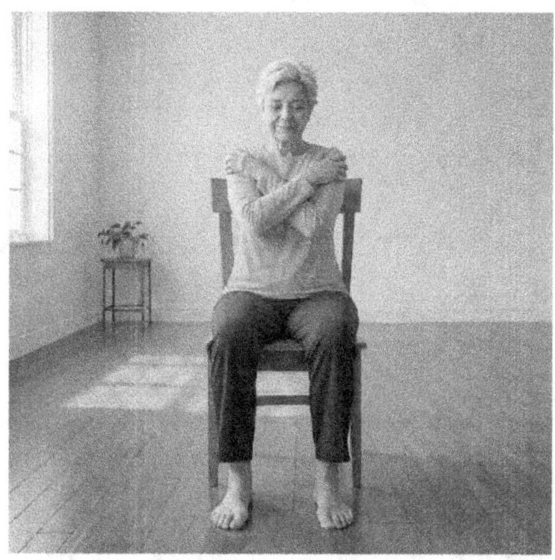

Release them back to the sides.

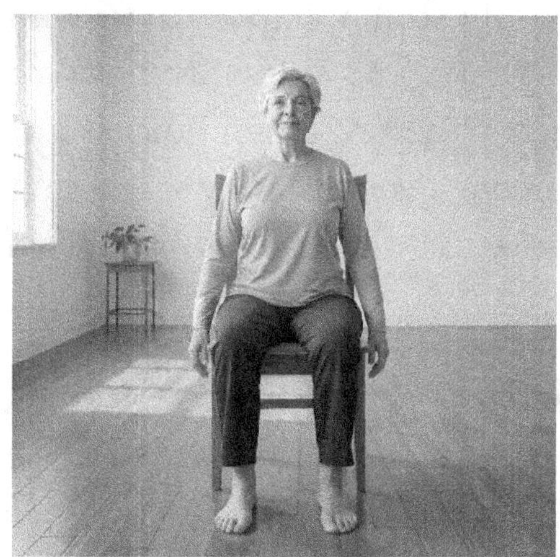

This closing movement, arms wrapping inward across the chest, stimulates the parasympathetic nervous system and creates a palpable contrast with the expansive opening of the inhale.

Repetitions: Four to six full cycles per session.

Modification: Those with limited shoulder range can perform a smaller arc, sweeping the arms only to chest height and keeping the crossing gesture at the abdomen rather than the chest.

6.3 Leg Raises and Hip Circles

Lower Body Mobility: A New Focus

Week 2 introduces the first movements specifically designed to mobilize the hip joint through its full circular range of motion. The Seated Leg Raise and Hip Circle build on the Knee Lifts and Leg Extensions from Chapter 4, but move beyond linear up-and-down or forward-and-back patterns to explore the full rotational capacity of the hip socket.

The hip joint is a ball-and-socket joint designed for multi-directional movement. In sedentary older adults, only a fraction of this range is used in daily life, and the unused portions progressively stiffen. Hip stiffness contributes directly to lower back pain, reduced gait quality, and difficulty with common activities such as sitting down and standing up, getting in and out of a car, and navigating stairs. Regular circular hip movement, even at a very small range, maintains the synovial fluid distribution and connective tissue pliability that the joint needs to remain functional and comfortable.

Movement 1: Seated Leg Raises

Purpose: To strengthen the hip flexors and quadriceps while improving controlled lower limb mobility.

Starting position: Sit upright, slightly forward on the seat. Hands rest lightly on the thighs or armrests. Feet flat on the floor.

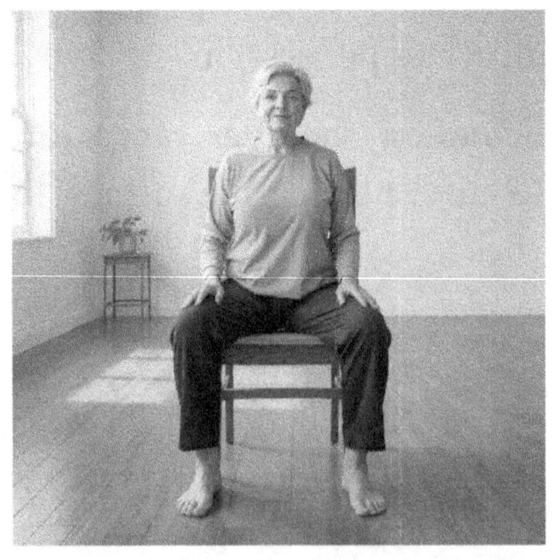

Step 1: Ground both feet. Take one breath. On the exhale, engage the lower abdomen gently.

Step 2: On the inhale, slowly raise the right leg, lifting the entire thigh off the seat and extending the leg forward and upward to a comfortable height. The foot can remain relaxed or gently flexed.

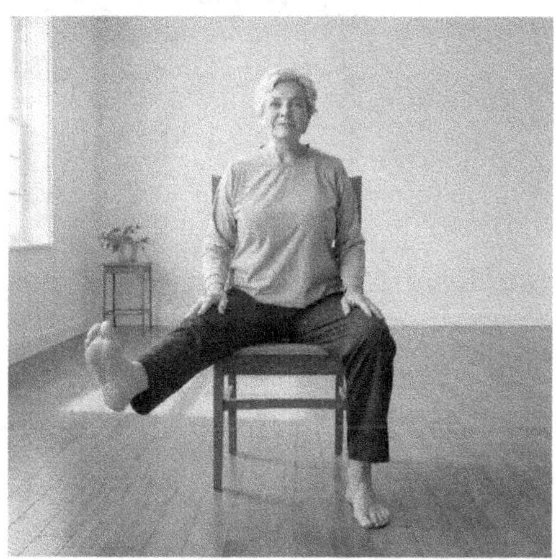

Step 3: Hold the raised position for one breath, maintaining the torso upright and the raised leg steady.

Step 4: On the exhale, slowly lower the right leg back to the floor with control.

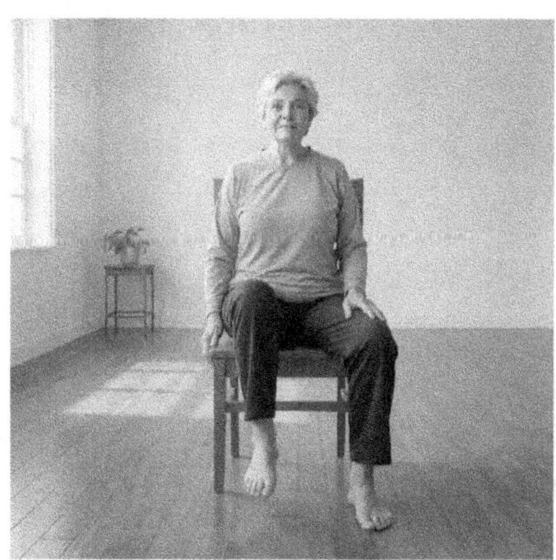

Alternate to the left leg. One cycle is one right raise and one left raise.

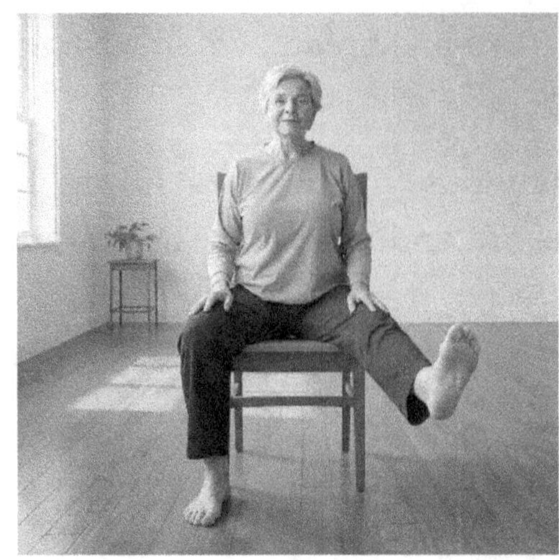

Repetitions: Three to five cycles alternating sides per session.

Modification: Those with hip replacement or significant hip arthritis should raise only the heel off the floor rather than the full thigh, maintaining the activation benefit without hip joint loading.

Movement 2: Seated Hip Circles

Purpose: To mobilize the hip joint through its full rotational range, distribute synovial fluid, and reduce stiffness in the hip flexors and external rotators.

Starting position: Sit upright, feet flat on the floor, hip-width apart. Hands rest lightly on the thighs.

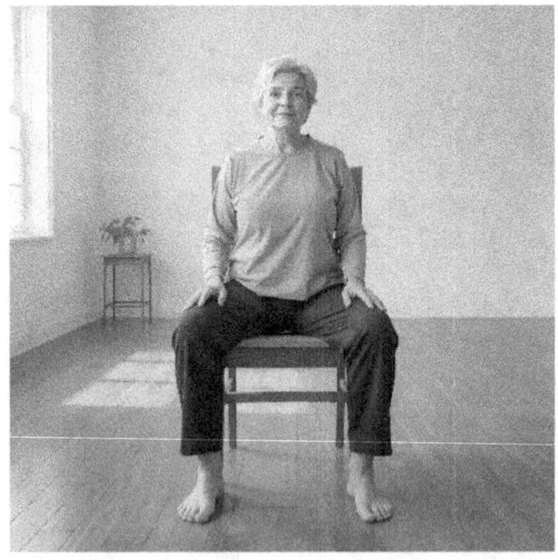

Step 1: Lift the right knee slightly off the seat, just enough to allow free rotation of the hip joint. The foot hangs loosely below the knee.

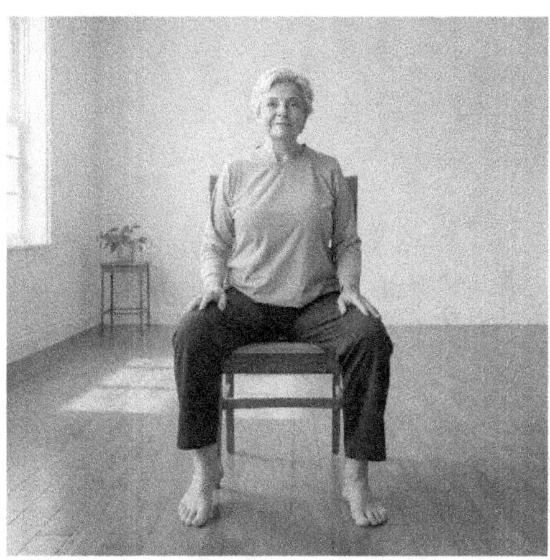

Step 2: Begin moving the raised right knee in a small, slow circle, rotating the hip joint. Move the knee outward to the right, then forward, then inward to the left, then back and around, completing the circle. Keep the movement small and comfortable in Week 2.

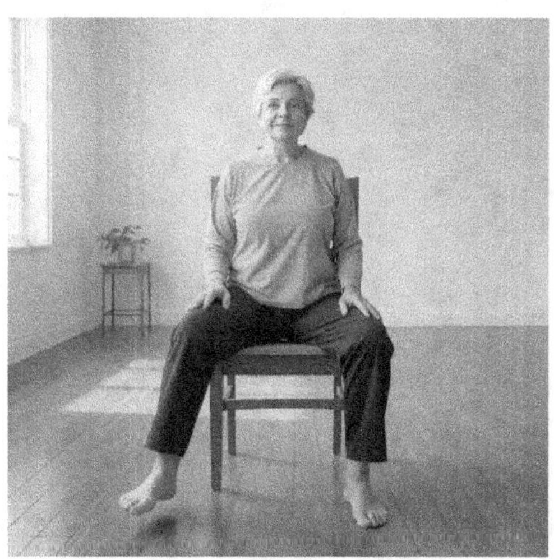

Step 3: Complete four slow circles in one direction.

Reverse for four circles in the opposite direction

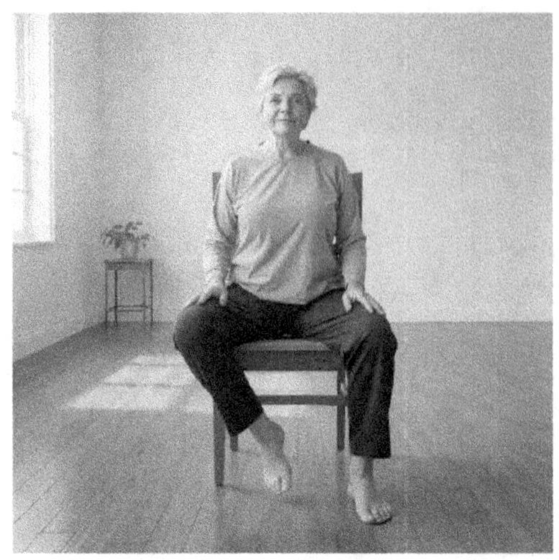

Lower the right foot gently back to the floor and repeat on the left side.

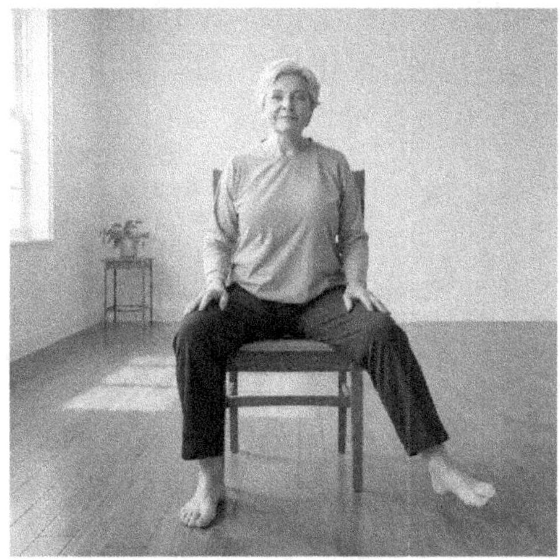

Repetitions: Four circles each direction on each side per session.

Modification: For very limited hip mobility, simply move the knee forward and back or side to side rather than in a full circle, gradually building toward the circular range over subsequent sessions.

6.4 Slow Side-to-Side Movements

Lateral Balance: Building the Foundation for Stability

The slow side-to-side movement is one of the most functionally important exercises in the entire program for fall prevention and daily balance confidence. It trains the body's ability to shift weight laterally in a controlled, conscious way, which is exactly what the body must do when navigating uneven terrain, stepping sideways to avoid an obstacle, or recovering from a moment of instability.

In standing balance, the ability to control a lateral weight shift is managed by the hip abductors, the gluteus medius in particular, along with the lateral core stabilizers and the ankle proprioceptors. In Chair Tai Chi, the seated version of this movement trains the same lateral control patterns from a safe, supported position where the consequences of any instability are completely eliminated.

Practiced consistently through Week 2 and beyond, this movement builds the neurological confidence for lateral stability that transfers directly to standing and walking.

Starting position: Sit upright, feet flat on the floor hip-width apart. Both hands rest lightly on the thighs. Spine lengthened.

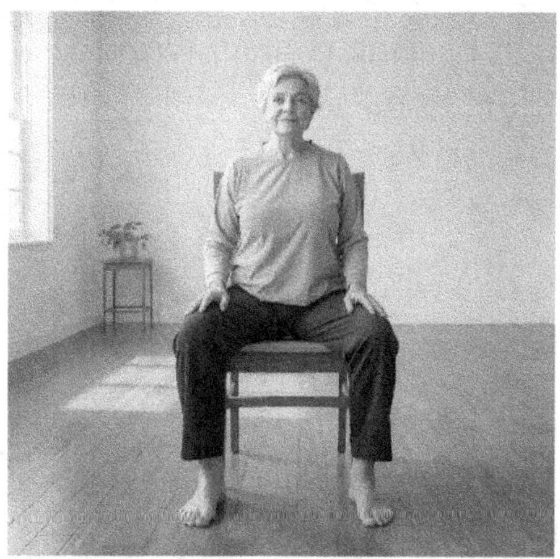

Step 1: Find Center

Take one full breath and feel your weight distributed evenly between the left and right sit bones. This centered, balanced starting position is the reference point you will return to with each repetition.

Step 2: Inhale and Shift Right

On your inhale, slowly allow your weight to shift to the right, leaning the upper body gently to the right while keeping both sit bones on the seat. The left sit bone will lighten slightly as the right one accepts more weight. Allow the right arm to float outward slightly from the thigh as the shift occurs.

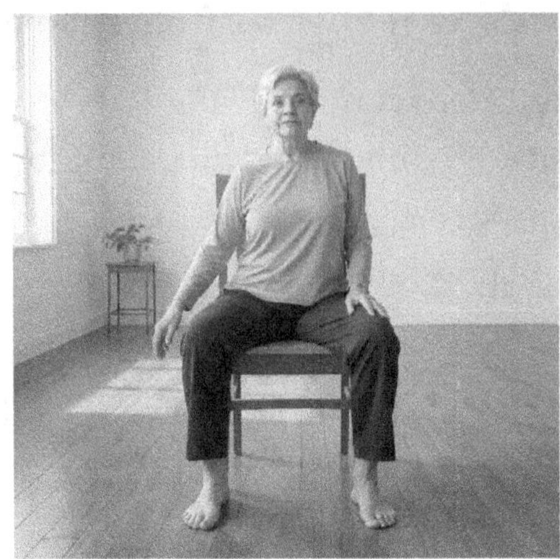

Step 3: Exhale and Return to Center

On the exhale, slowly bring the body back to the centered position. Feel both sit bones return to equal weight-bearing contact with the seat. Pause for one natural breath at center before shifting to the left.

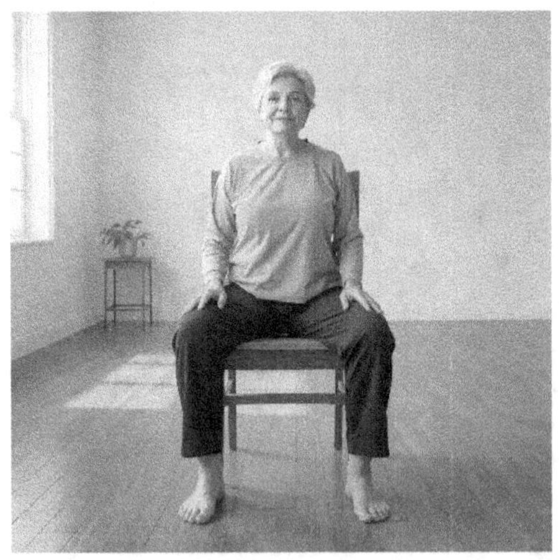

Step 4: Inhale and Shift Left

On your next inhale, mirror the movement to the left. Allow the weight to shift to the left sit bone, the upper body inclines gently left, and the left arm floats slightly outward.

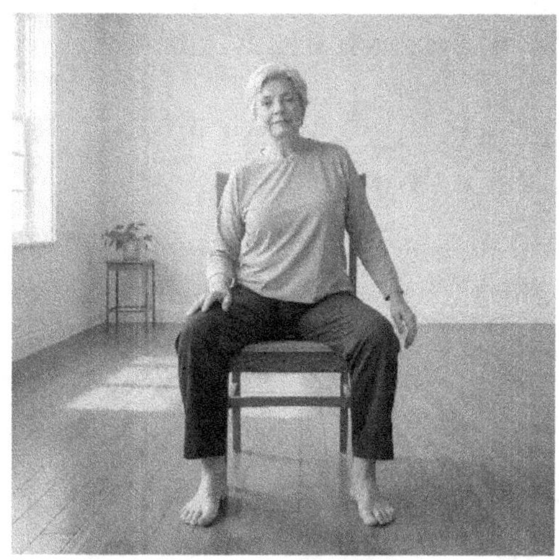

Exhale to return to center.

Repetitions: Four to six full side-to-side cycles per session.

Advanced variation: As the body shifts to one side, extend the opposite arm upward in a diagonal reach, combining the lateral weight shift with an upper body reach for a more integrated whole-body movement.

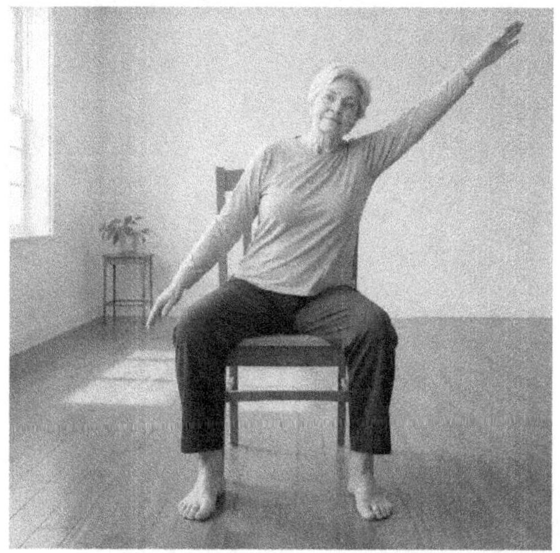

Modification: Those who feel any discomfort in the lower back during the shift should reduce the range of the incline to a very subtle weight shift, barely perceptible, and build gradually over the week.

Closing Week 2: What Mobility Actually Means

By the end of this week, you will have added four new movement categories to your practice: spinal rotation through the Seated Twists, chest and shoulder opening through the Breath and Reach, hip joint mobility through the Leg Raises and Hip Circles, and lateral balance training through the Side-to-Side Movements.

None of these movements require flexibility you do not currently have. They require only the willingness to move through the range that is available to you today, with patience, with breath, and with the understanding that range comes with practice, not with force.

Mobility is not a physical characteristic you either have or do not have. It is a quality your body generates through regular, intelligent movement. Every session this week is a small but genuine investment in a body that moves more freely, more confidently, and with less discomfort than it did seven days ago.

Week 3 will build on everything you have developed in these two weeks and introduce the flowing, connected sequences that begin to feel like traditional Tai Chi form.

Chapter 7: Week 3 — Strengthening and Coordination

Two weeks in, your body has changed more than you may realize. The movements that felt unfamiliar in Week 1 are now recognizable. The breath coordination that required deliberate effort in Week 2 is beginning to happen more naturally. Your joints are moving through ranges they had not visited in some time, and the ten minutes you give to this practice each day has begun to feel less like a task and more like something you genuinely look forward to.

Week 3 builds on all of that. This week the practice shifts its center of gravity from learning and loosening toward strengthening and coordinating. The movements introduced here are more complex, requiring the upper and lower body to work together in integrated patterns. They draw more deeply on focus and intention. And they begin to feel, unmistakably, like Tai Chi.

Approach this week with confidence. You have earned it.

7.1 Seated Cloud Hands

The Movement That Defines Tai Chi

If there is one movement that captures the essence of Tai Chi more completely than any other, it is Cloud Hands, known in Chinese as Yun Shou. It appears in virtually every Tai Chi style and form. It is described in classical Tai Chi texts as the movement that embodies the art's fundamental principles most completely: continuous flow, the absence of force, the coordination of the entire body through the waist, and the quality of soft, unhurried attention that makes Tai Chi different from every other movement practice.

In its standing version, Cloud Hands involves shifting weight side to side while the arms rotate in large, overlapping arcs. In the seated version, the weight shift becomes a gentle lateral lean, and the arms move in the same slow, circular, overlapping pattern. The result is a movement that looks like the hands are parting the air in slow, horizontal circles, or drawing through clouds.

The benefits are substantial: Cloud Hands develops rotational coordination between the two sides of the body, trains the nervous system's ability to manage two independently moving limbs simultaneously, deepens the breath-movement connection, and produces a quality of meditative calm that students consistently describe as one of the most pleasurable experiences in the entire practice.

Starting position: Sit upright, feet flat on the floor hip-width apart. Both hands rest loosely in the lap, palms facing upward. Spine lengthened.

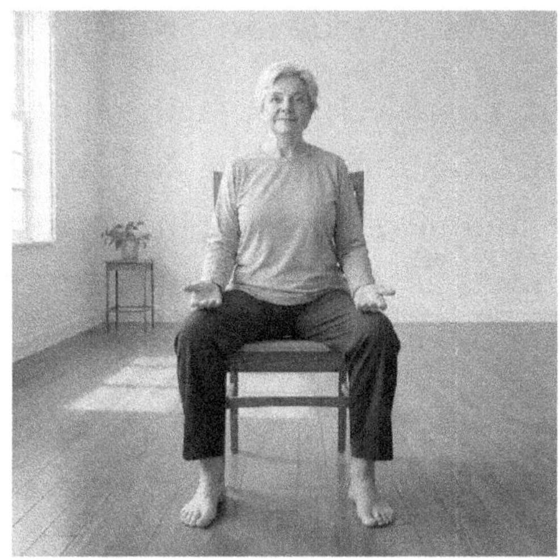

Step 1: Raise Both Hands to Center

Lift both hands to chest level, palms facing inward toward the body, right hand slightly higher than left, with the hands separated by about twelve inches. This is the beginning position of Cloud Hands.

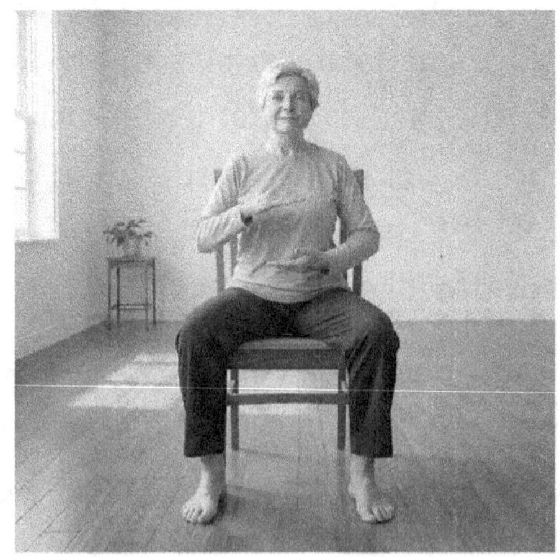

Step 2: Begin the Rotation, Right Hand Rising

As you inhale, gently turn your waist and upper body just a few inches to the right. Let your arms travel with your torso. As you turn, let your right hand naturally floats up toward face level, while your left hand gently presses down toward your lap. Keep your elbows soft and relaxed.

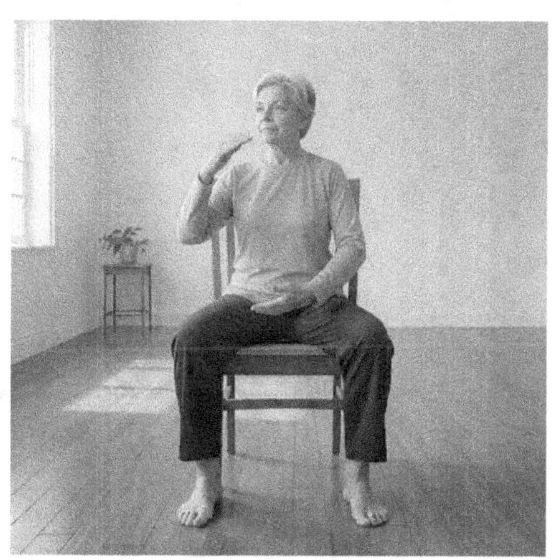

Step 3: The Right-Side Midpoint

Finish your gentle turn to the right. Your torso is now facing slightly right. Your right hand is high (near your face) and your left hand is low (near your left hip), both palms still facing you. Do not pause or freeze here; Tai Chi is like a slowly turning wheel that never entirely stops.

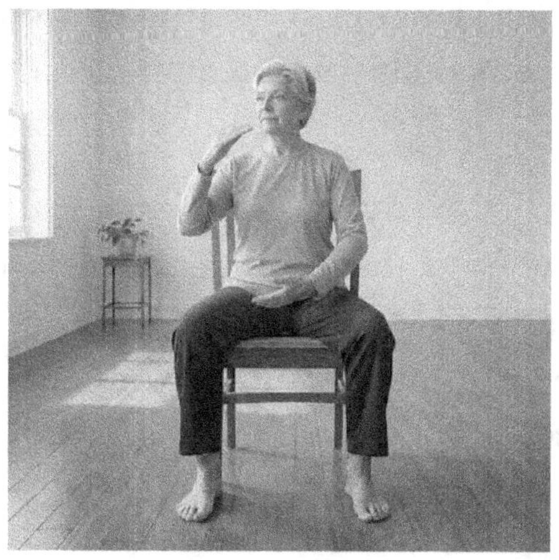

Step 4: Reverse, Left Hand Rising

As you slowly exhale, begin turning your waist back through the center and over to the left. As your body turns, your hands elegantly trade places: your left hand floats up toward your face, while your right hand presses softly down toward your lap. Let the hands pass each other in front of your chest like passing clouds.

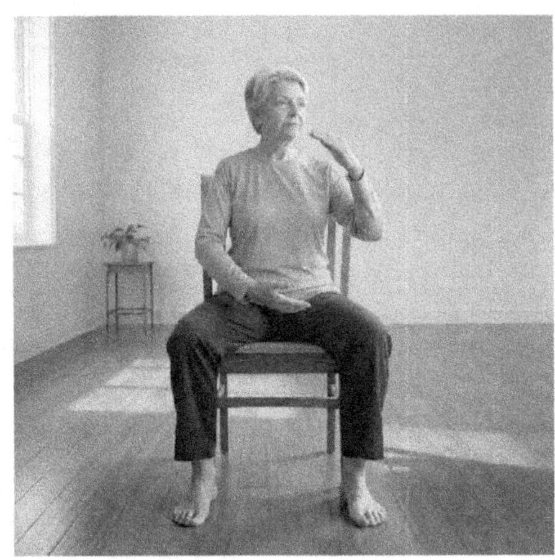

Step 5: Establish the Continuous Flow

After two or three individual rotations on each side, allow the movement to become fully continuous, one seamless cycle flowing into the next without any identifiable beginning or end point. Add a very gentle lateral body sway to accompany each arm's rise, leaning very slightly right when the right hand is high, leaning very slightly left when the left hand is high.

Repetitions: Complete six to eight full cycles (three to four rotations on each side). Move only as fast as your breath. If your breathing is slow, your hands should be slow.

Modification: If reaching up toward your face causes any pinching or discomfort in your shoulders, simply lower the movement. Keep your "high" hand at chest level, and your "low" hand near your lap. The magic of Tai Chi comes from the gentle turning of the waist, not how high you can lift your arms. Keep it comfortable, and keep it yours.

7.2 Knee Lifts and Arm Strokes

Integrating Upper and Lower Body

The Knee Lift and Arm Stroke is the first movement in this program to fully integrate upper and lower body in a coordinated, simultaneous pattern. It builds on the Knee Lifts from Chapter 4 and the Arm Swings and Push movements from the same chapter, combining them into a single flowing sequence that requires the brain and nervous system to coordinate opposite-side arm and leg movements.

This cross-body integration is one of the most powerful neurological training tools available to older adults. It activates the corpus callosum, the neural bridge between the brain's two hemispheres, and has been associated in research with improvements in processing speed, reaction time, and motor coordination that transfer directly to balance and gait quality in daily life.

Starting position: Sit upright, feet flat on the floor hip-width apart. Both hands rest on the thighs. Spine lengthened.

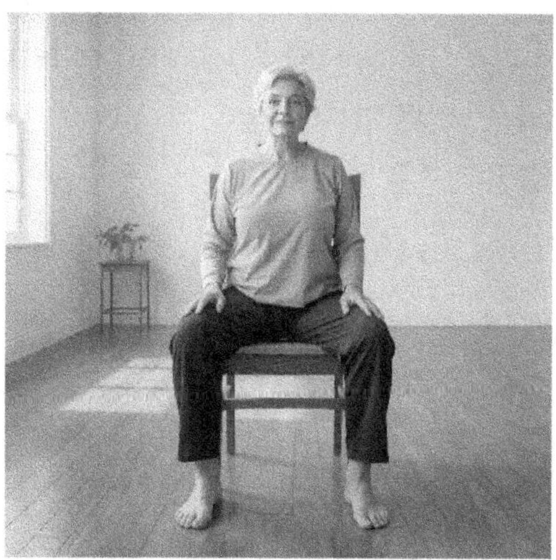

Step 1: Root and Prepare

Take one full breath cycle. On the exhale, feel both feet grounded and both sit bones anchored. Let the arms be loose and heavy in the lap.

Step 2: Lift Right Knee, Stroke Left Arm Forward

On your inhale, simultaneously lift the right knee upward while sweeping the left arm forward and upward in a long, smooth stroke from the hip to just above shoulder height. The right arm moves gently back and slightly outward as the left moves forward, mirroring natural walking opposition.

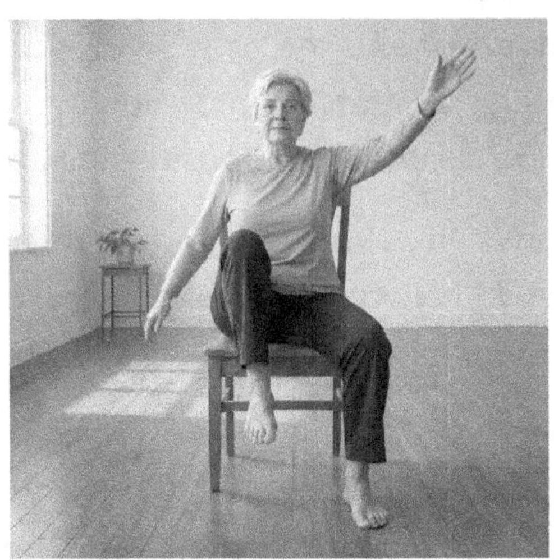

Step 3: Hold Briefly at the Peak

At the peak of the inhale, hold the raised knee and extended arm position for one natural breath pause. Feel the coordinated engagement through the core, the raised hip flexor, and the extended shoulder.

Step 4: Lower and Transition on the Exhale

On the exhale, simultaneously lower the right knee back to the floor and draw the left arm back toward the hip.

Without pausing, transition smoothly to the opposite side: left knee rises as the right arm strokes forward and upward.

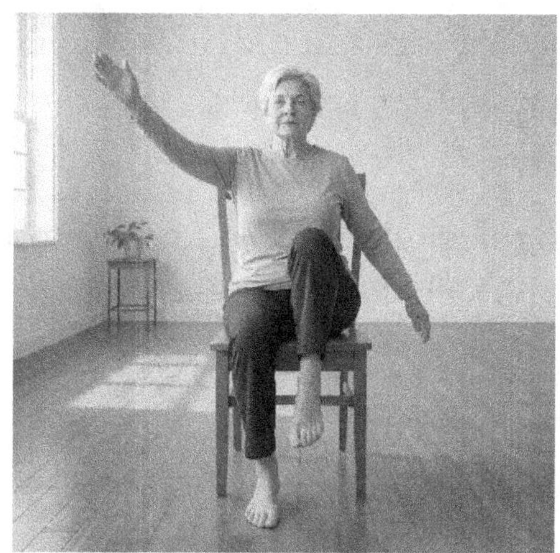

Repetitions: Four to six full cycles alternating sides per session.

Modification: You can perform the knee lift and arm stroke as two separate sequential movements rather than simultaneously, building toward the integrated version over the course of the week.

7.3 Golden Rooster Stand

Seated Balance Mastery

The Golden Rooster Stand is one of the most celebrated postures in all of Tai Chi. In its traditional standing form, it involves balancing on one leg with the opposite knee raised and the arms in a specific position, a posture that demands exquisite balance and focused, rooted attention.taoistwellness+1

The seated adaptation for Chair Tai Chi preserves the most important training element of the original posture: the single-leg rooting combined with the upward energy of the raised limb. Rather than standing on one leg, you ground through one foot with complete intention while the other leg rises. The result is a movement that simultaneously trains hip flexor strength, postural stability, focused attention, and the quality of rooted presence that is the defining characteristic of the Golden Rooster in all its forms.

Research and classical Chinese medicine practitioners both note that single-leg balance training, even in a seated and supported form, activates the six major meridians that pass through the legs and provides significant neurological benefits including improved coordination, reduced fall risk, and enhanced spatial awareness.

Starting position: Sit upright, slightly forward on the seat. Both feet flat on the floor, hip-width apart. Arms hang loosely at the sides or rest on the thighs.

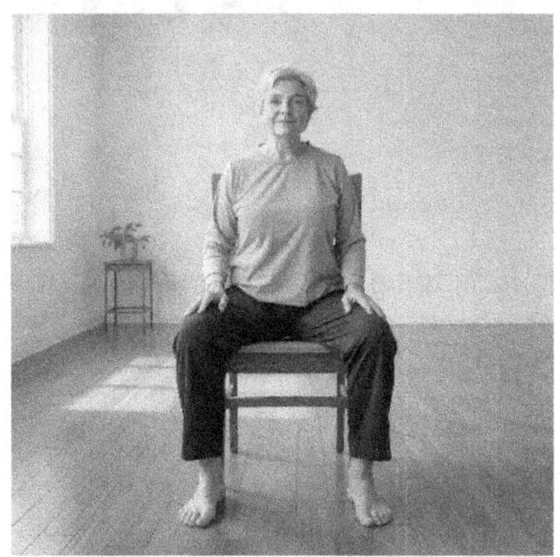

Step 1: Find Your Root

Ground the left foot firmly and completely into the floor, as though the foot is the root of a tree pressing down through the earth. Take one breath. With each exhale, feel the left foot becoming more grounded and more anchored.

Step 2: Rise, Right Arm and Right Knee Together

On your inhale, simultaneously raise the right arm upward, elbow bent, hand rising toward face level with the palm facing inward, while lifting the right knee upward in the Knee Lift pattern. The left foot remains completely and firmly grounded as the single point of lower body contact. This coordinated rise of the right arm and right knee is the defining gesture of the Golden Rooster.

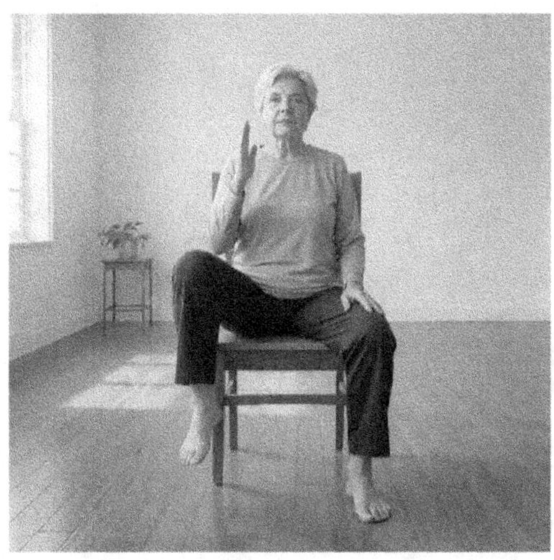

Step 3: Hold with Complete Attention

Hold the raised position for three to five full breath cycles. The quality of attention during the hold is the practice itself. Feel the rootedness of the grounded left foot. Feel the upward energy of the raised right arm and knee. Notice the core engagement that maintains the posture without gripping or tension.

Step 4: Lower with Control

On an exhale, slowly lower both the right arm and the right knee simultaneously, returning the foot to the floor and the arm to the resting position.

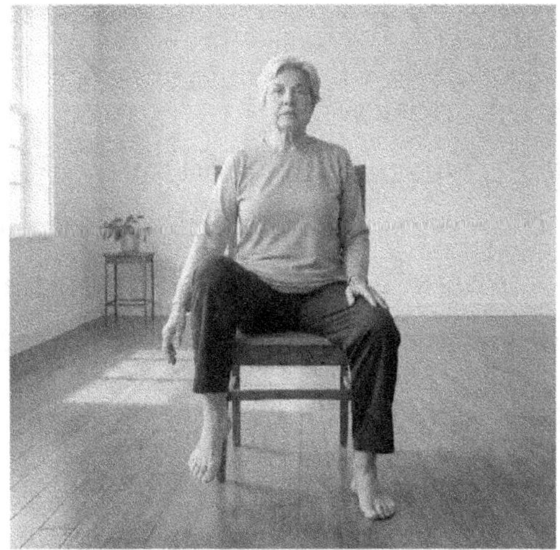

Take one full breath at center before beginning on the left side.

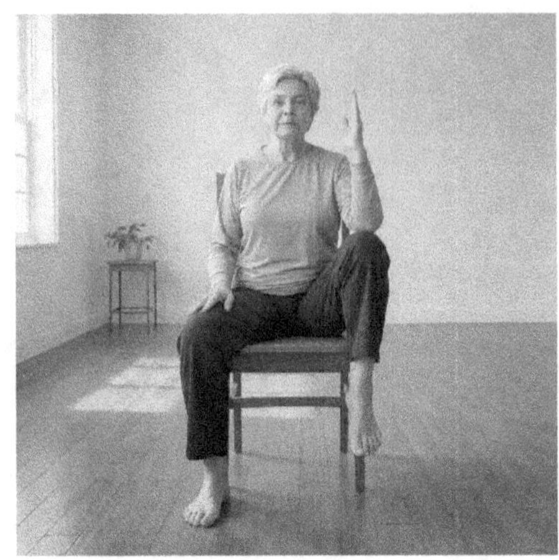

Repetitions: Two to three holds on each side per session, progressively increasing the hold duration across the week.

Modification: For those with limited hip flexor strength, raise only the heel off the floor while the arm rises, maintaining the coordinated arm-leg gesture at a reduced range.

7.4 Chair Tai Chi Brush Knee

A Classic Form Adapted for the Chair

The Brush Knee is one of the most widely recognized movements in traditional Tai Chi forms, appearing in Yang, Chen, and Sun style lineages. It describes a gesture in which one hand sweeps downward across the knee in a brushing arc while the opposite hand pushes forward, combining a downward clearing movement with a forward issuing of energy in a single coordinated gesture.

In the seated version, the pushing arm and the brushing arm remain the defining elements, while the lower body participation shifts from the weight-bearing step of the standing form to a coordinated engagement of the opposite knee and thigh. The result is a movement that develops upper and lower body coordination, lateral flexibility through the torso, and the flowing integration of opposites, one arm moving down and inward while the other moves forward, that is the hallmark of Tai Chi's bilateral intelligence.

Starting position: Sit upright, feet flat on the floor hip-width apart. Both hands rest in the lap. Spine lengthened.

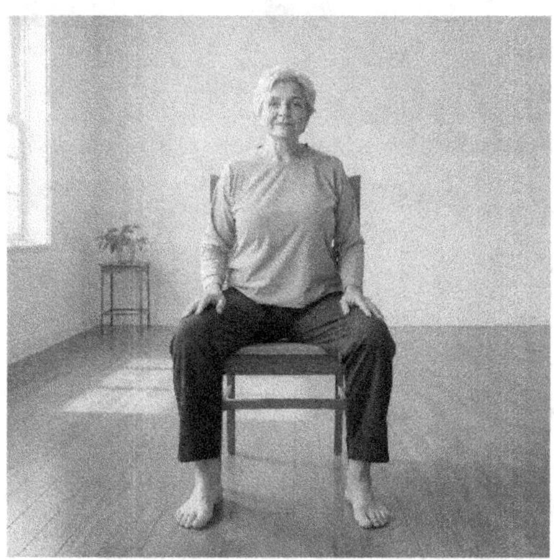

Step 1: Gather the Right Hand to the Ear

On your inhale, slowly raise the right hand upward and back toward the right ear, palm facing forward, elbow pointing outward. This is the gathering position from which the push will originate. Simultaneously, let the left hand rest on the left thigh, ready to brush.

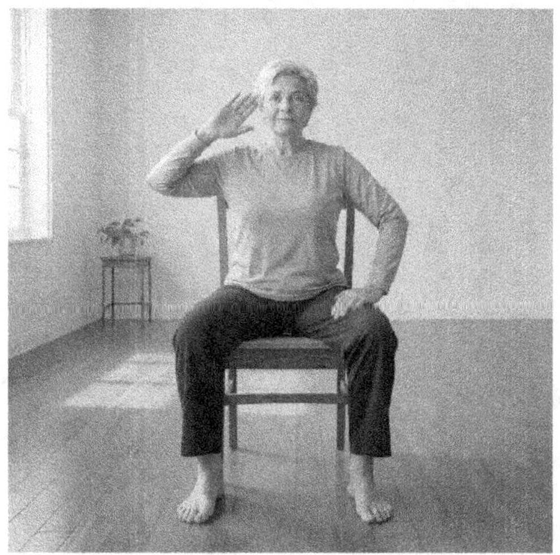

Step 2: Brush Left Hand Across the Left Knee

On the exhale, sweep the left hand downward and across the left knee in a smooth brushing arc, as though clearing something from the knee. The palm faces downward throughout the brush. The movement is controlled and intentional, a clean arc from thigh to beyond the knee.

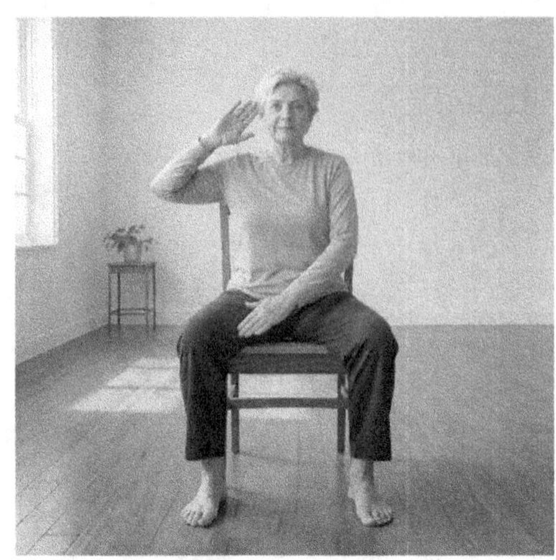

Step 3: Push the Right Hand Forward

Simultaneously with the brushing arc of the left hand, push the right hand forward from the ear toward the front of the body, extending the arm forward at chest level with the palm facing forward. The push and the brush complete together at the end of the exhale, the right arm extended forward and the left hand having completed its arc below and beyond the left knee.

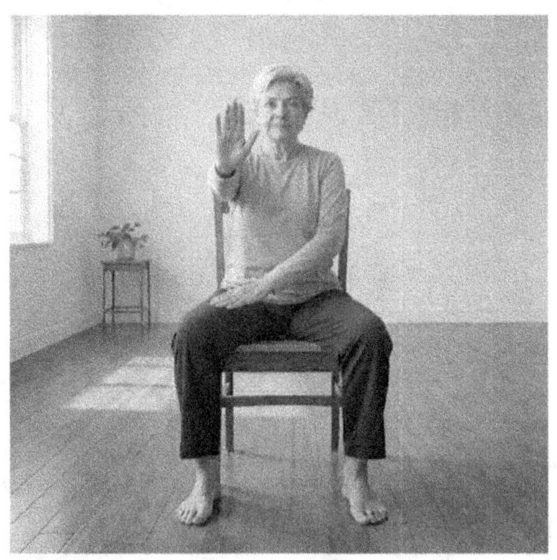

Step 4: Reset and Alternate Sides

On the next inhale, draw the right hand back to resting and raise the left hand toward the left ear for the gathering position.

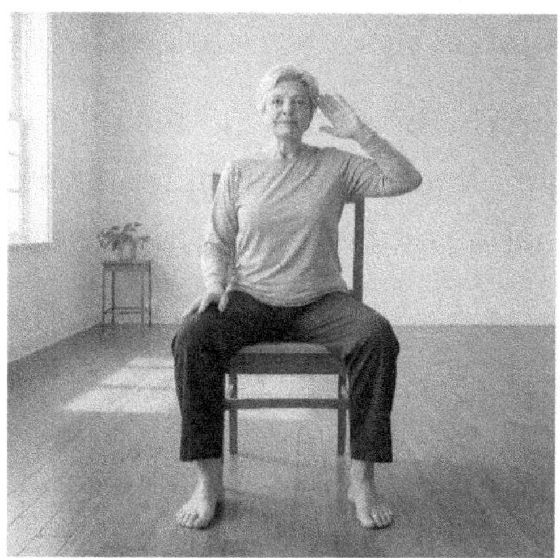

Exhale and brush the right hand across the left knee

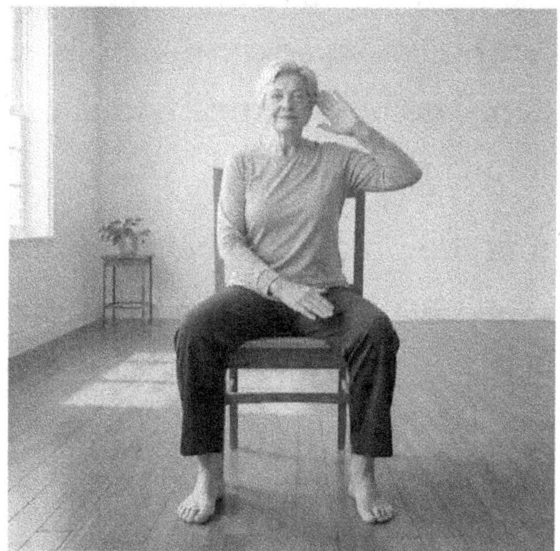

Push the left hand forward.

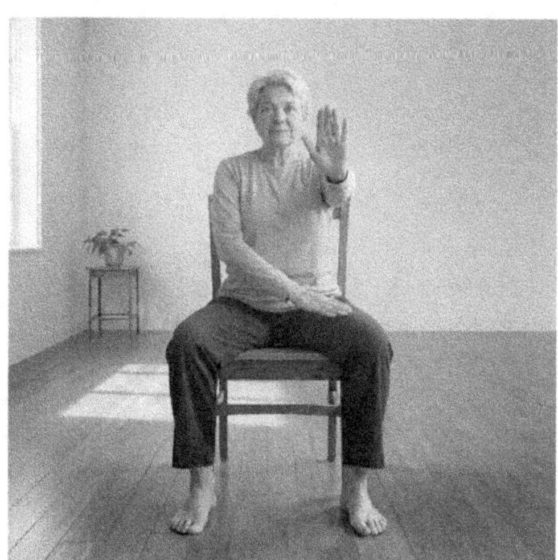

One full cycle is the Brush Knee on both sides.

Repetitions: Three to four full cycles alternating sides per session.

Modification: You can perform the brush and the push as two separate sequential movements rather than simultaneously, completing the brush before beginning the push, until the coordination of the combined movement develops naturally.

Closing Week 3: The Shift You Will Feel

Somewhere in this week, possibly as early as the second or third session, you will notice that something has changed in how your practice feels. The movements are no longer procedures you are executing. They are beginning to be something you inhabit. The Cloud Hands sequence will begin to feel genuinely fluid. The Golden Rooster will surprise you with how steady you can become in a position that felt precarious in the first session. The Brush Knee will click into a coordinated whole at a moment you cannot predict and cannot force.

This is the shift from learning the practice to being in the practice. It is what Week 3 is designed to produce. And once it arrives, even briefly, it will give you a clear, felt sense of what this practice is capable of offering over the months and years ahead.

Chapter 8: Week 4 — Fluidity and Mental Focus

You are in the final week of this four-week program. Take a moment, before you read further, to acknowledge what that means. Four weeks ago, you were reading Chapter 1 and deciding whether this practice was really for you. Now you have a daily habit. You have a practice space. You have a body that moves differently than it did when you started, more freely, more deliberately, with more awareness and less apprehension.

Week 4 is not the end. It is the beginning of something more sustained. This week the emphasis shifts from building new movements to deepening the quality of everything you already know. The movements this week may feel familiar, but the way you will be asked to inhabit them is new. Fluidity, mental focus, visualization, and honest reflection on your own progress are the themes of Week 4.

Move slowly this week. Breathe fully. Pay close attention. This is where the practice becomes a practice.

8.1 Seated Leg Extensions with Flow

Familiar Movement, Deepened Quality

The Seated Leg Extension was first introduced in Chapter 3 as a foundational lower body exercise and revisited in Chapter 4 as part of the core movement vocabulary. By Week 4, the physical mechanics of the movement are familiar. This section does not re-teach the movement. It asks you to do something more demanding: perform a movement you already know with a quality of fluid, unhurried attention that makes it feel entirely different from its earliest versions.

In Week 4, the Leg Extension becomes part of a flowing lower body sequence that moves from one leg to the other without pausing at the center, creating a continuous alternating rhythm that resembles the lower body component of the Seated Tai Chi Walk from Chapter 4 but with fuller extension and deeper breath integration.

Starting position: Sit upright, slightly forward on the seat. Hands rest lightly on the thighs or armrests. Feet flat, hip-width apart.

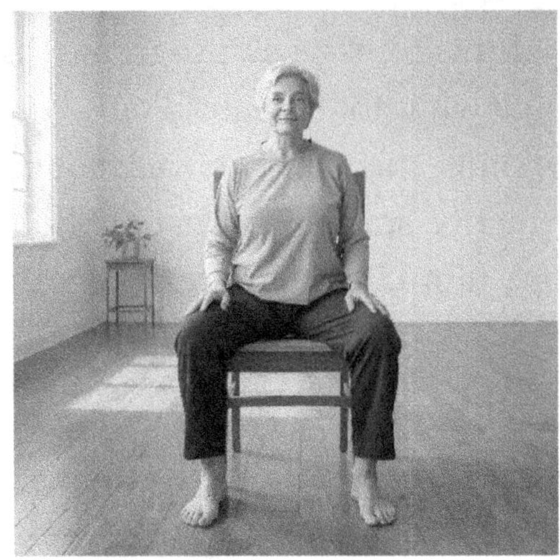

Step 1: Begin with Grounded Breath

Take two full breath cycles before beginning. On the second exhale, let the hands become completely heavy and relaxed on the thighs. Feel the distinction between the quality of rest in this moment and the quality of movement that is about to begin.

Step 2: Slide and Extend the Right Leg on the Inhale

On your inhale, slide the right foot forward along the floor and extend the right leg out to a comfortable full extension, foot gently flexed, toes pointing upward. The extension should reach its full comfortable length by the time the inhale is complete.

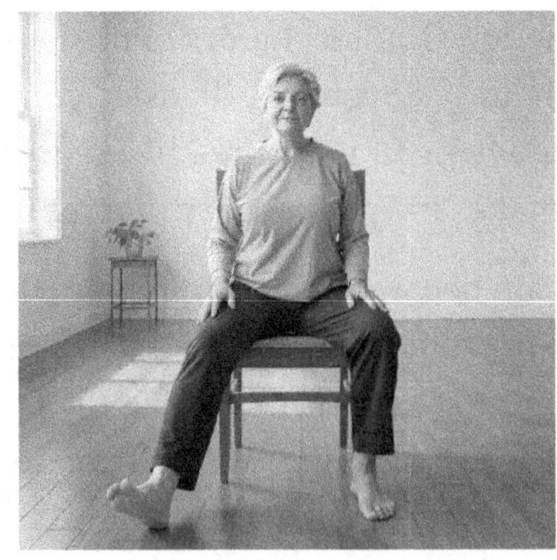

Step 3: Transition Without Pausing

Rather than returning to the starting position before extending the left leg, begin returning the right leg on the exhale while simultaneously beginning the left leg's extension. The goal is a flowing, continuous alternation, the right leg returning as the left extends, creating a smooth, wavelike lower body movement.

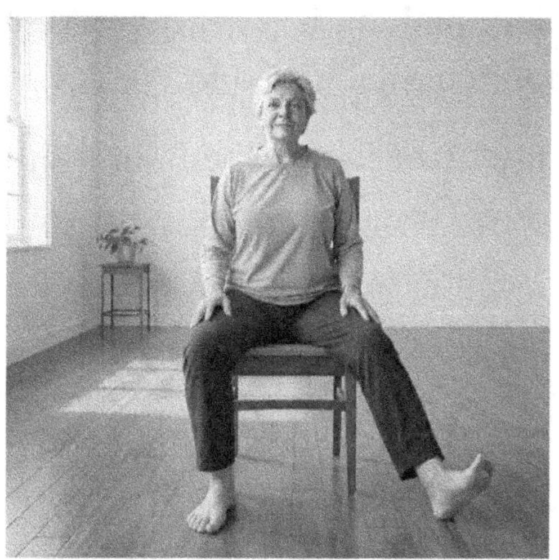

Step 4: Find the Flow Rhythm

After four to six alternations, allow the movement to settle into a continuous rhythm in which the breath, the leg extensions, and the transitions all occur as part of one uninterrupted flow. The movement should feel like a continuous, gentle tide, alternating from side to side with no abrupt stops or starts.

Repetitions: Eight to ten full alternating cycles per session.

Modification: For those who find continuous alternation too demanding, return to the complete stop-and-reset pattern from Chapter 3 and simply bring greater breath integration and intention to the familiar movement.

8.2 Tai Chi Push Movements for Flow

From Mechanics to Expression

The Tai Chi Push was introduced in Chapter 4 as a bilateral forward press executed with breath coordination and whole-body intention. By Week 4, the physical pattern is established. This section develops the Push into a flowing, multi-directional sequence that moves through forward, upward, and downward pushes in a single continuous gesture, creating a more complex and expressive movement that embodies Tai Chi's principle of continuous, uninterrupted flow.

The addition of directional variation in Week 4 requires greater proprioceptive awareness and coordination, making it a genuine Week 4 challenge that builds meaningfully on the foundation established in Week 1.

Starting position: Sit upright, feet flat on the floor. Both hands gathered at chest level, palms facing forward, fingers pointing upward. The familiar starting position from Chapter 4.

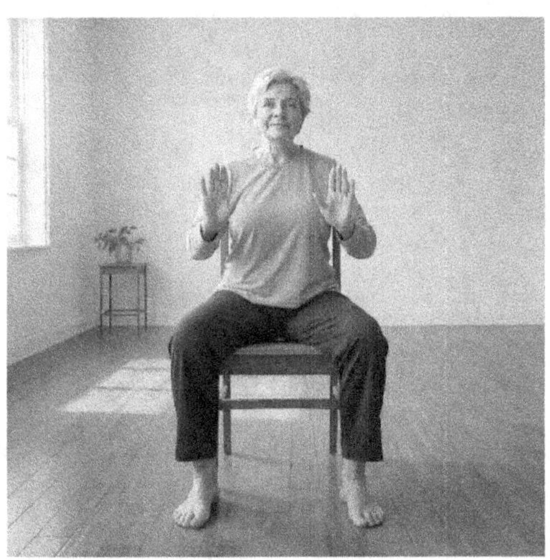

Step 1: Forward Push on the Exhale

Begin with the familiar forward push from Chapter 4. On the exhale, extend both arms forward to comfortable full extension, palms facing forward, elbows gently soft.

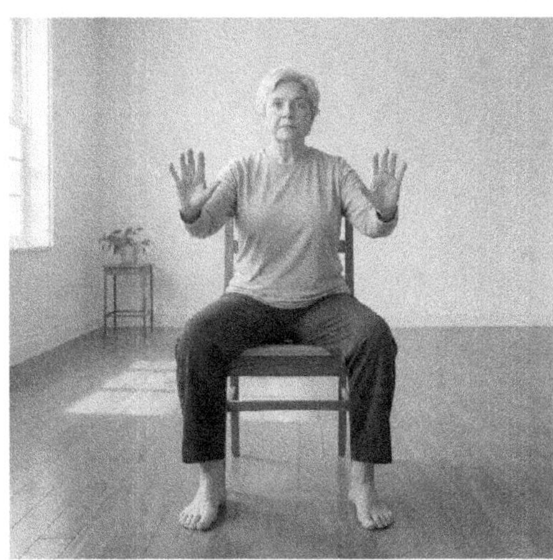

Step 2: Transition to Upward Push on the Inhale

Without returning to the gathered position, on the inhale rotate both wrists so the palms face upward and draw the arms slightly back while raising them upward, transitioning from the forward push into an upward lifting gesture. The arms rise from chest level to slightly above, as though lifting something from below.

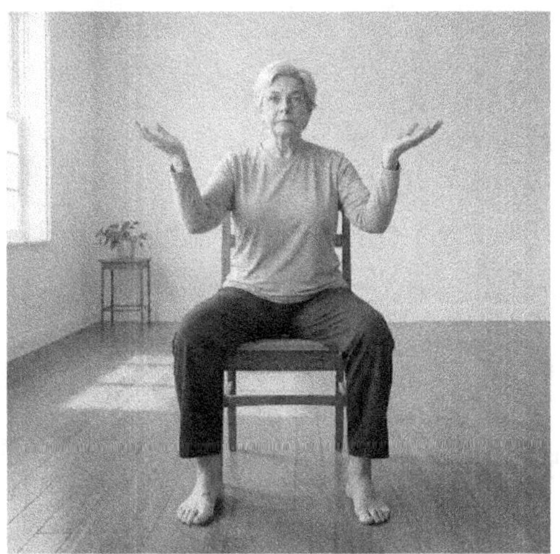

Step 3: Press Downward on the Exhale

On the exhale, rotate the wrists again so the palms face downward and slowly press both hands downward from the elevated position back toward hip level, as though pressing something gently downward toward the ground. This downward press completes the three-directional push sequence.

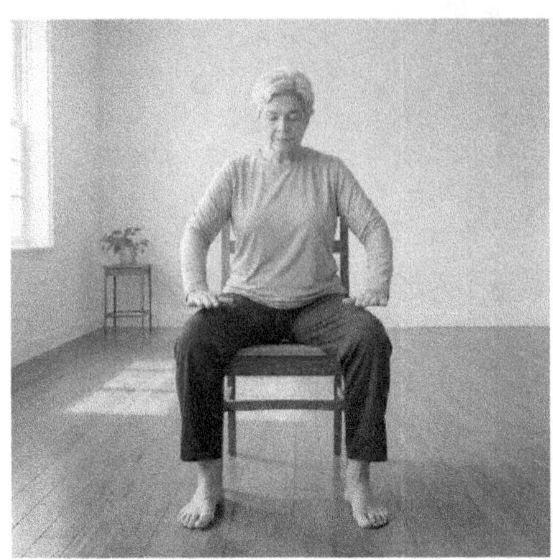

Step 4: Return and Cycle

On the next inhale, draw both hands back upward and inward to the gathered chest position and begin the three-directional sequence again: forward push, upward lift, downward press. Allow the transitions between the three directions to become progressively smoother until the entire sequence flows as one uninterrupted gesture.

Repetitions: Four to six full three-directional cycles per session.

Modification: Those who find the three-directional sequence too complex can continue with the single forward push from Chapter 4 with added intention and flow, building toward the full sequence over successive sessions.

8.3 Visualization and Mental Clarity Practices

The Inner Dimension of Practice

Throughout this program, the emphasis has been on the physical dimensions of Chair Tai Chi: the movements, the breath, the posture, the specific health benefits for joints and circulation and balance. All of that is real and important. But in Week 4, we turn attention fully toward the dimension that Tai Chi practitioners have always considered equally important: the inner landscape of the practice.

Visualization in Tai Chi is not imagination for its own sake. It is a practical tool for improving movement quality, deepening the relaxation response, and cultivating the quality of mental clarity that seniors consistently report as one of the most valuable outcomes of regular practice. When you visualize the internal experience of a movement rather than simply executing it mechanically, the nervous system engages more completely, muscle recruitment patterns improve, and the calming effects of the practice deepen significantly.

The following three visualization practices are designed to be used during or immediately after your regular movement sessions. They require no additional time and no special ability. They require only attention.

Visualization Practice 1: The Warm River

Use this during Cloud Hands or any flowing arm movement.

As your arms move through their circular arcs, imagine that your hands are moving through a warm, slowly flowing river. Feel the gentle resistance of the water, not as an obstacle but as a substance that gives your movement depth and texture. Notice how imagining this resistance slightly slows the movement and deepens the quality of the arm-path through space. Allow the warmth of the imagined water to spread from the hands into the wrists, forearms, and shoulders. Stay with this image through four to six complete movement cycles.

Visualization Practice 2: The Rooted Tree

Use this during the Golden Rooster Stand or any single-leg balance work.

Before and during the held balance position, close your eyes for one breath cycle and imagine that your grounded foot has roots extending downward through the floor, through the foundation of the building, and deep into the earth below. Feel the stability that comes from imagining this rootedness. Notice how the quality of the balance changes when the nervous system is given this specific mental image of groundedness. The more vivid and specific the image, the more the body responds.

Visualization Practice 3: Moving Through Light

Use this as a closing practice at the end of any session.

At the end of your session, let the hands rest in the lap and close the eyes. Take three slow breath cycles. With each inhale, imagine drawing clear, bright light into the body through the top of the head. With each exhale, imagine that light spreading through the chest, the arms, the lower back, the legs, all the way to the feet. After three cycles, simply sit in the quality of illuminated, relaxed presence for thirty to sixty seconds before opening the eyes.

Students who practice this closing visualization regularly report that it extends the calming effects of the session significantly into the hours that follow, and that over several weeks, it begins to produce a baseline quality of mental clarity that persists throughout the day.

8.4 Evaluating Your Progress

Looking Back With Clear Eyes

Let's take a moment to look back. Be honest with yourself, not critical, just honest. Think about that first day. How did your shoulders feel then versus now? Can you reach for a coffee mug with a little less stiffness? These small wins are what we're counting.

Read through the following areas of reflection and take a few minutes either mentally or in writing to note your honest responses.

Physical mobility. Think back to Day 1, when you sat in your practice chair for the first time and attempted the Arm Swings from Chapter 3. How did your shoulders feel then? How do they feel now? Can you raise your arms to shoulder height with greater ease? Has the range of the Side Reach increased? Is the Seated Forward Bend deeper than it was in Week 1?

You do not need to measure these changes precisely. Simply notice them. Many students find that the improvements are most visible in activities outside of practice: reaching for something on a high shelf without hesitation, turning to look behind them without stiffness, getting up from a chair with noticeably less effort than four weeks ago.

Balance and coordination. Has the Golden Rooster Hold become more stable across the week? Does the Seated Tai Chi Walk feel more naturally coordinated? Have you noticed any change in how you navigate everyday situations that require balance, such as stepping over a threshold, walking on uneven ground, or shifting your weight to reach for something?

Breath and relaxation. Does diaphragmatic breathing feel natural now, or does it still require conscious effort? Have you noticed any change in your general stress level, sleep quality, or ability to calm yourself in moments of anxiety? Have there been moments during the day, outside of practice, when you noticed yourself breathing more slowly and fully than you used to?

Mental clarity. Many students notice this dimension of progress before they notice the physical changes. Has your focus improved? Do you feel a cleaner quality of mental alertness in the hours following your morning practice? Have you noticed any change in memory, mood, or the general sense of cognitive ease that your days carry?

What you want to continue. Week 4 ends but your practice does not have to. Which movements have become genuinely enjoyable? Which benefits matter most to you personally? The answers to these questions are the raw material from which your ongoing, post-program practice will be shaped.

Take your time with this reflection. What you find here is not a report on your adequacy. It is a map of genuine, earned progress, and the beginning of understanding what this practice is growing into for you.

Chapter 9: Chair Tai Chi for Specific Health Needs

A four-week program of Chair Tai Chi produces general health benefits that will serve almost every senior who completes it. But the practice is also flexible enough to be specifically adapted for particular health conditions that many older adults live with every day. This chapter addresses three of the most common: arthritis, cardiovascular health concerns, and cognitive challenges. Each section offers targeted guidance on which movements to emphasize, how to modify them for the condition in question, and what the research and clinical evidence say about the specific benefits available.

If you live with one of these conditions, this chapter is not a medical consultation. It is a companion to your medical care, offering you information you can bring to your healthcare team and movement tools that complement rather than replace professional treatment.

9.1 For Arthritis Relief

Understanding the Relationship Between Arthritis and Movement

Arthritis is not one condition but a family of them. Osteoarthritis, the most common form in older adults, involves the gradual wearing of joint cartilage, leading to pain, stiffness, and reduced range of motion, primarily in the knees, hips, hands, and spine. Rheumatoid arthritis is an autoimmune condition that produces inflammation in the joint lining, affecting joints throughout the body and creating periods of painful flare alternating with relative remission.

In both forms, the instinct is often to protect the painful joint by moving it less. This instinct is understandable but counterproductive over time. Joints need movement to maintain the distribution of synovial fluid, the joint's natural lubricant. They need the gentle load of movement to stimulate the cartilage cells that maintain the joint surface. And the muscles around the joint, when they weaken from disuse, provide less support to the joint, which then experiences more stress with every movement. Immobility feeds arthritis pain rather than relieving it.

Chair Tai Chi addresses this cycle directly. Its movements are slow enough to avoid inflammatory stress, varied enough to take each joint through its natural range, and consistent enough to maintain the joint health benefits that only regular movement can provide.

Most Beneficial Movements for Arthritis

Seated Arm Circles are among the most targeted exercises available for shoulder and elbow arthritis. With both arms raised to a comfortable height, make slow, small circles in the horizontal plane, as though stirring something gently. Begin with circles no larger than a tennis ball and gradually expand to dinner-plate size as the joint warms. The rotational movement distributes synovial fluid throughout the entire shoulder socket, reducing the stiffness that peaks after periods of rest.

Wrist Flexions and Circles from the Chapter 5 warm-up are particularly valuable for osteoarthritis of the hand and wrist, one of the most functionally limiting forms of arthritis for older adults. Performed twice daily, before and after the main practice session, they reduce morning stiffness significantly over two to three weeks of consistent practice.

Seated Knee Lifts from Chapter 4, performed at a small, comfortable range, maintain the quadriceps strength that protects the knee joint from the grinding that occurs when the muscles are weak. The key for knee arthritis is to keep the range within the pain-free zone strictly, any movement that produces sharp or worsening joint pain should be reduced in range or discontinued until the joint is assessed.

Cloud Hands from Chapter 7 provides continuous, flowing movement through the shoulder, elbow, and wrist joints simultaneously, making it one of the most efficient arthritis management tools in the entire program.

An older student in one of my retirement community classes had been managing severe hand osteoarthritis for eleven years when she joined the Chair Tai Chi program. She had been told by her rheumatologist to keep the hands moving but had found most hand exercises too painful or too boring to maintain. After six weeks of daily practice that included Wrist Flexions and Cloud Hands, she reported a significant reduction in morning stiffness, from approximately ninety minutes to under thirty minutes, and her grip strength measurably improved at her next occupational therapy appointment. Her therapist incorporated Chair Tai Chi into her formal treatment plan as a result.

A Note on Flare Days

On days when arthritis symptoms are acutely elevated, do not push through practice at the normal intensity. Instead, perform only the Breath and Posture Check-In from Chapter 5 and the visualization practices from Chapter 8. The parasympathetic activation of slow breathing reduces systemic inflammation at the hormonal level and provides meaningful relief even when physical movement is not appropriate. The practice continues on flare days. It simply takes a different form.

9.2 For Heart Health and Circulation

Tai Chi as Cardiovascular Medicine

The evidence supporting Tai Chi as a beneficial practice for cardiovascular health is among the most robust in the entire field of integrative medicine. A comprehensive 2021 systematic review published in the *European Journal of Preventive Cardiology* found that regular Tai Chi practice was associated with significant reductions in systolic and diastolic blood pressure, reductions in resting heart rate, improvements in heart rate variability, and reduced markers of systemic inflammation, all independent of other lifestyle factors.

Chair Tai Chi specifically benefits cardiovascular health through three primary mechanisms. First, the continuous, low-intensity movement maintains an elevated level of peripheral circulation compared to complete rest, stimulating blood flow to the extremities and reducing the venous pooling that contributes to the swollen ankles, cold feet, and circulatory discomfort common in sedentary older adults.

Second, the diaphragmatic breathing practiced in every session functions as an auxiliary cardiovascular pump. Each full breath cycle creates changes in intrathoracic pressure that assist the return of blood to the heart. Over a ten-minute session this effect is cumulative and meaningful, particularly for those with reduced cardiac output from age-related changes or mild heart failure.

Third, the consistent activation of the parasympathetic nervous system through breath and mindful movement directly counteracts the elevated sympathetic tone, the chronic low-grade stress response; that is one of the primary drivers of hypertension and cardiovascular disease in older adults.

Most Beneficial Movements for Cardiovascular Health

Seated Leg Raises/Curls are one of the most effective circulation exercises available for the lower limbs. Sitting upright, slowly curl the right heel back toward the chair leg by bending the knee, then straighten and repeat on the left. The alternating contraction and release of the hamstring muscles acts as a muscular pump for venous blood return from the lower legs, directly addressing the circulatory stagnation that contributes to varicose veins, leg swelling, and the discomfort of peripheral vascular disease. Perform ten to fifteen slow alternating curls as an addition to the regular warm-up.

Arm Strokes from Chapter 7 engage the large muscle groups of the shoulder girdle and upper back in slow, repetitive movement that maintains a gentle but sustained elevation of heart rate and significantly improves upper body circulation.

The Tai Chi Push from Chapters 4 and 8 engages both the pushing and returning phases to work the pectoral and posterior shoulder muscles in a smooth, rhythmic alternation that sustains circulation while remaining well within the cardiovascular comfort zone of even those with significant cardiac limitations.

Full-body breathing practices, particularly the three-to-one exhale-to-inhale ratio described in Chapter 3, reduce blood pressure measurably during practice and have been shown in multiple studies to produce lasting reductions in resting blood pressure in older adults who practice consistently over eight to twelve weeks.

A retired teacher in her mid-seventies attended her first Chair Tai Chi class at her cardiologist's suggestion after a mild cardiac event. She began with the simplest movements, Arm Swings and slow breathing, practiced daily for twelve minutes each morning. At her three-month cardiac follow-up, her resting blood pressure had decreased from an average of 148/92 to 131/81, a reduction her cardiologist described as clinically significant. She continued the practice and maintained that improvement at her six-month follow-up.

Working Within Cardiac Limitations

If you have a diagnosed cardiac condition, work closely with your cardiologist or cardiac rehabilitation team when using this program. Most cardiac patients can practice Chair Tai Chi safely at all stages of recovery, but specific movement intensity recommendations may need to be individualized. Rate of perceived exertion should remain low throughout, no movement in this program should cause breathlessness, chest discomfort, or heart pounding. If any of these symptoms occur, stop immediately and contact your healthcare provider.

9.3 For Cognitive Decline and Brain Health

Why Tai Chi Is Uniquely Positioned to Help

Most exercise helps the brain in one way: it gets more blood flowing up there. That's valuable, but Tai Chi does something extra.. Tai Chi offers that benefit and several others simultaneously, which is why it stands apart from virtually every other movement practice in its demonstrated effects on cognition.

A landmark NIA-funded study published in the *Annals of Internal Medicine* studied 304 adults aged 65 and older with mild cognitive impairment across six months of regular Tai Chi practice. The traditional Tai Chi group raised cognitive test scores by 1.5 points compared to a stretching-only control group. A cognitively enhanced version of Tai Chi, which added mental challenges during movement, raised scores by nearly three points, a clinically meaningful improvement that no pharmaceutical intervention for mild cognitive impairment has consistently matched.

A systematic review in *BMC Geriatrics* confirmed that Tai Chi practice spanning twelve weeks to one year produced small to moderate but clinically relevant enhancements in overall cognitive functioning in elderly individuals with cognitive impairment, compared to both non-intervention and active control groups. Additional research published in *JAMA Network Open* found that Tai Chi outperformed fitness walking in improving global cognitive function in older adults with mild cognitive impairment over thirty-six weeks of practice.

The reasons are physiological and neurological simultaneously. Tai Chi increases cerebral blood flow through its aerobic component. It has been shown in neuroimaging studies to strengthen the hippocampus, the brain region most critical for memory formation and most vulnerable to Alzheimer's-related degeneration. It activates the prefrontal cortex through the demands of learning, sequencing, and remembering movement patterns. And the bilateral, cross-body coordination that defines movements like Cloud Hands and the Seated Tai Chi Walk directly stimulates the corpus callosum, the neural bridge between the brain's hemispheres whose health is strongly associated with cognitive resilience in older age.

Importantly, Chair Tai Chi addresses these mechanisms even in its gentlest, most accessible form. The brain benefits do not require vigorous aerobic intensity. They require consistent engagement of movement, breath, attention, and memory, all of which are built into every session of this program from Week 1 forward.

How Cognitive Challenges Change the Practice

Seniors experiencing cognitive decline range from those with mild memory complaints who are otherwise fully independent to those with moderate dementia who require significant daily support. Chair Tai Chi can be adapted meaningfully across this entire spectrum, though the adaptation looks quite different at each level.

For those with **mild cognitive impairment**, the standard four-week program in this book is appropriate with minimal modification. The primary adaptation is to reduce the complexity of multi-step movement instructions during the learning phase and to use more repetition before introducing new movements. Establishing a completely consistent daily practice environment, the same chair, the same space, the same time, the same opening breath sequence, is especially important, as environmental cues compensate for the reduced reliability of prospective memory in mild impairment.

For those with **moderate cognitive challenges**, simplify the practice to three to four core movements rather than the full repertoire, and use consistent verbal cues that remain identical session to session. The goal is not variety or progression but the reliable, daily repetition of a small number of known movements that the brain and body can enter without the cognitive overhead of learning something new. Cloud Hands, the Breath and Posture Check-In, Arm Swings, and the closing visualization from Chapter 8 form an excellent simplified core practice for this population.

For those in the **early stages of dementia**, the practice should be led or guided by a caregiver or family member rather than self-directed. Dr. Paul Lam's research at the Tai Chi for Health Institute has developed specific protocols for Alzheimer's and dementia populations, and his principle is directly applicable here: the goal is quality time in movement and breath, not performance of specific forms. Any movement that the person can make with some degree of attention and breath awareness constitutes a valid and beneficial practice.

Most Beneficial Movements for Cognitive Health

Cloud Hands from Chapter 7 is the single most cognitively engaging movement in this program. It requires simultaneous management of two independently moving limbs, coordination of body rotation with arm movement, and maintenance of a flowing rhythm, all while following the breath. The bilateral coordination demand is precisely the kind of neural challenge that researchers have identified as most beneficial for preserving and improving cognitive function. Practice Cloud Hands as long as it feels comfortable in each session. For cognitive health purposes, more repetitions of Cloud Hands are more valuable than a wider variety of shorter-duration movements.

The Seated Tai Chi Walk from Chapter 4 trains the cross-body neural pathways through alternating opposite-arm-opposite-leg coordination. This is the same type of bilateral patterning used in cognitively enhanced Tai Chi research programs and has been directly associated in studies with improved dual-task performance, the ability to manage two mental or physical tasks simultaneously, which is one of the cognitive functions that declines earliest and most functionally disruptively in normal aging and mild cognitive impairment.

The Brush Knee from Chapter 7 adds the cognitive demand of sequencing, the need to remember which hand brushes and which pushes, and which side comes next, making it a useful working memory exercise embedded within physical practice.

Adding Cognitive Challenges to Any Movement is a technique directly supported by NIA-funded research. During any sustained movement sequence, a caregiver, practice partner, or the practitioner themselves can introduce simple concurrent mental tasks to elevate the cognitive training effect:

- Count backward from twenty by twos during Cloud Hands

- Name a fruit, vegetable, or animal with each alternating step of the Seated Tai Chi Walk

- Spell a four or five-letter word aloud, one letter per breath cycle, during Arm Swings

- Recall a specific memory, a person's face, a place from the past, and describe it mentally in detail during the closing visualization

These additions do not complicate the physical practice. They overlay it with exactly the kind of dual-task neural demand that research has shown to produce the most significant cognitive improvements.

The Emotional Dimension of Cognitive Decline

Cognitive decline carries an emotional weight that must be acknowledged honestly in any guide that addresses it. Fear of further decline, grief about lost abilities, frustration with the inconsistency of memory, and the social isolation that often accompanies cognitive challenges are not peripheral concerns. They are central to the experience of living with cognitive impairment, and they are dimensions of health that Chair Tai Chi addresses alongside the neurological ones.

The calming, rhythmic quality of regular practice consistently reduces anxiety and agitation in cognitively impaired populations, including those with moderate dementia. The physical engagement provides a reliable source of embodied wellbeing on days when memory and cognition are unreliable. And the social experience of practicing with a caregiver, family member, or group provides the kind of positive relational engagement that neuroscientists now recognize as one of the most powerful protective factors against cognitive deterioration available to older adults.

A caregiver whose husband was diagnosed with early Alzheimer's disease began practicing Chair Tai Chi alongside him, three mornings each week as a shared activity. She reported that within two months his agitation in the late morning, a common symptom in early Alzheimer's, had reduced noticeably on practice days. His neurologist noted that his engagement and responsiveness during appointments was visibly different. She continued the practice and described it as the most consistently positive part of their day together.

Practical Notes for Caregivers and Family Members

If you are supporting a senior with cognitive challenges through this program, the following principles will help you make the practice sustainable and genuinely beneficial:

- **Keep every session identical in structure.** The opening breath check-in, the same two or three movements, and the closing visualization, in the same order, every time. Predictability is not monotony for someone with cognitive impairment. It is safety.

- **Use calm, consistent verbal cues.** Speak slowly, use the same words for the same movements every session, and allow longer pauses after instructions. Cognitive processing speed is reduced in impairment and the practice should never feel rushed.

- **Follow the person's lead on duration.** Ten minutes is a guide, not a rule. Some sessions will be four minutes. Some, on particularly good days, may extend to fifteen. Let engagement and comfort set the pace rather than the clock.

- **Celebrate every session.** Not performance, not correct form, not measurable improvement. Simply the showing up, the breathing, and the moving together. That is the whole point, and it is more than enough.

Chapter 10: Continuing Your Journey with Chair Tai Chi

You have completed the four-week program. The movements that were new are now known. The habit that was fragile is now established. The body that arrived at this practice four weeks ago is not quite the same body that has arrived at this final chapter.

What comes next is entirely yours to define. This chapter offers guidance for the path forward, specific, practical, and grounded in the same respect for where you actually are that has guided every page of this book.

10.1 Integrating Tai Chi into Daily Life

From Program to Practice

The most important transition in any wellness journey is the one from following a structured program to maintaining an organic, self-directed practice. Programs have beginnings and endings. Practices do not. A practice is simply something you do because it is part of how you live, as natural and unconditional as eating or sleeping.

Getting there requires a shift in how you think about Chair Tai Chi. Rather than something you do for thirty days and then evaluate, it becomes something you do the way you drink your morning tea or call a friend on Sunday afternoons, habitually, comfortably, without needing to decide to do it each time.

The following practical strategies will help you make that transition.

Anchor to an existing habit. The most reliable way to sustain any new behavior is to attach it to one that is already automatic. Practice Chair Tai Chi immediately after your morning coffee, or immediately before your afternoon rest, or in the first ten minutes after dinner. Let the existing habit pull the new one along.

Keep your chair in place. The physical cue of your practice chair in its designated spot is a more powerful motivator than any intention. When the chair is visible and ready, the practice feels accessible. When you have to set it up, the friction of preparation becomes a reason not to start.

Use the movements outside of formal practice. Cloud Hands can be practiced at a dining table while a kettle boils. Wrist circles can be done during any period of seated rest. The Breath and Posture Check-In can be used at any moment during the day when stress or discomfort arises. Tai Chi is not only a practice you do in a dedicated session. It is a vocabulary of movement and breath that can be woven through the entire fabric of your day.

Set a minimum. On difficult days, when energy is low or motivation has temporarily retreated, commit to a minimum of three minutes rather than the full ten. Three minutes of breathing and simple arm movements is not the full practice, but it maintains the neurological habit and keeps the chain of consecutive practice days unbroken. More often than not, three minutes leads to ten.

10.2 Staying Motivated

The Honest Reality of Long-Term Practice

No one maintains any practice with equal enthusiasm across weeks and months and years. Motivation fluctuates. Life intervenes. There will be days when ten minutes feels like too much, weeks when illness or travel or difficult circumstances break the routine, and moments when you genuinely cannot remember why you started.

These are not failures of character. They are the normal rhythms of a human life. The seniors who maintain Chair Tai Chi for years are not the ones who feel consistently motivated. They are the ones who have developed practical strategies for returning to the practice after it has lapsed, without self-judgment and without the need to start from the beginning.

Track your practice with a simple journal. A small notebook kept near the practice chair, used for nothing more than a date and one sentence after each session, "Felt stiff but finished" or "Good session, shoulder looser today," creates a visible record of effort that becomes genuinely motivating over time. Looking back at thirty or sixty entries and seeing the accumulated consistency is more motivating than any external encouragement.

Connect with others. Chair Tai Chi classes are available in most communities through senior centers, YMCAs, recreation departments, and many hospital wellness programs. Practicing with others adds social connection, accountability, and the specific pleasure of moving in synchronized rhythm with other people, an experience that produces measurable increases in the bonding hormone oxytocin and significantly improves practice enjoyment and retention.

Celebrate non-performance wins. A win in this practice is not a new flexibility record or an impressively held balance posture. A win is showing up on a day when you did not feel like it. A win is noticing that you slept better. A win is the comment from a family member that you seem more relaxed lately. Honor these. They are the actual currency of progress in Chair Tai Chi.

Refresh the practice periodically. After several months, if the practice begins to feel too routine, add one new movement or sequence, explore a different Tai Chi video online, attend one community class, or revisit an early chapter of this book with fresh eyes. The practice has more depth than any program can fully cover. There is always somewhere new to go within it.

A 78-year-old woman who has been practicing Chair Tai Chi for four years told me recently that the practice had become, in her own words, "the most reliable thing in my life." Not because it was always enjoyable, but because it was always there, accessible, non-judgmental, and genuinely responsive to how she felt on any given day. She had missed weeks during illness, traveled for months without a formal chair, and gone through periods of grief that made any physical practice feel meaningless. Each time she returned, the practice received her exactly as she was, and gave her back, a little at a time, the steadiness she had come to rely on it for.

10.3 Progress Tracking and Celebrating Milestones

Making Progress Visible

Progress in Chair Tai Chi is often gradual enough that it can be difficult to perceive from the inside of the experience. This is partly because the practice meets you where you are and improves from there, so the baseline shifts with the improvement and the gap between current and past capacity becomes invisible. Tracking progress creates the external record that makes the gap visible again and provides the encouragement that subjective experience sometimes cannot.

The following simple tracking approach requires no special tools, only the small journal described in the previous section.

Weekly physical notes. At the end of each week, take two minutes to write three brief observations about physical changes. Note one thing that feels easier than it did the week before. Note one movement that has improved in range or fluency. Note one area of chronic discomfort that has changed, either diminished or simply become more manageable.

Monthly mobility checks. Once a month, perform the following simple self-assessments and note the results. How high can you raise your arms without discomfort? How far can you turn your head to each side? How many seconds can you hold the Golden Rooster position on each side? Can you reach your hands further forward in the Seated Forward Bend than last month? These are not competitions. They are benchmarks that make invisible progress visible.

Consecutive practice day tracking. Mark each practice day on a simple calendar. The visual pattern of consecutive marked days is one of the most powerful motivators available, and the strong desire to not break a streak once established is a well-documented psychological phenomenon that works reliably in favor of consistent practice.

Celebrating milestones. Mark specific milestones with genuine acknowledgment. Completing the four-week program is a milestone worth celebrating. Reaching thirty consecutive practice days is a significant achievement. Noticing a specific physical improvement, sleeping through the night for the first time in months, walking to the mailbox without hip pain, turning to look over your shoulder without stiffness, these are the milestones that matter most, and they deserve to be recognized with the same warmth you would offer a friend who had accomplished something meaningful.

Because they are meaningful. The commitment you have made to your own health and wellbeing over these four weeks is an act of genuine self-respect. The improvements you have earned are the body's honest response to that respect.

The Practice Continues

There is one final thing worth saying as this book draws toward its close.

Chair Tai Chi has been practiced, in various forms, for centuries. The principles it is built on, the coordination of breath and movement, the cultivation of rooted attention, the understanding that slow is not the same as weak and that gentle is not the same as ineffective, are not trends or temporary wellness solutions. They are deep, tested, cross-cultural truths about what the human body and mind need in order to function well across the full length of a life.

You have spent four weeks touching the surface of something genuinely ancient and genuinely alive. The practice is not complete at the end of this book. In the Tai Chi tradition, the practice is never complete. It simply deepens, session by session, year by year, as long as you show up for it.

Show up. Move gently. Breathe fully. The practice will do the rest.

A Small Request

If this book made a difference for you, even in a small way, would you consider leaving an honest review on Amazon or through the website you got a hold of this book?

As an independent author, I don't have the marketing budget of large publishing houses. Reviews are how readers discover books like this. Your feedback truly helps this work reach others who may need it.

It only takes a minute, and your honest thoughts, positive or critical are genuinely appreciated.

Thank you for reading and for your support.

Closing Remark

There is something worth naming before you close this book and set it on the shelf or the side table or wherever it has lived beside your practice chair these past weeks.

Most people who pick up a health and wellness book read the first chapter, feel genuinely motivated, intend to return, and never do. You did not do that. You showed up. Day after day, in a chair in whatever room you chose, with whatever body you arrived with on any given morning, you moved. You breathed. You paid attention. That is not a small thing. In a world that rewards the dramatic and the extreme, ten quiet minutes of gentle, intentional movement every day is a quietly radical act.

Chair Tai Chi does not promise transformation overnight. It never has. What it promises, and what centuries of practice and decades of modern research have confirmed, is this: consistent, gentle, mindful movement changes the body. It changes the nervous system. Over time, it changes the way you inhabit your life.

You may have started this program because your balance was unsteady, or your joints ached in the morning, or your mind felt foggier than it used to. You may have started because someone you trust suggested it, or because something in Chapter 1 felt true in a way that made you want to try. Whatever brought you here, you stayed. And that matters.

What you have built across these ten chapters is not just a four-week exercise program. You have built a vocabulary of movement that belongs to you now. The Arm Swings, the Cloud Hands, the Golden Rooster Stand, the slow coordinated breath that accompanies every gesture, these are yours. They live in your body. They will be easier to return to than they were to learn, because the nervous system holds what it has practiced, even through weeks of absence, even through illness or travel or the interruptions that life brings without asking permission.

The practice does not require you to be well. It does not require you to be pain-free, or strong, or flexible, or certain. It only requires that you sit down, take a breath, and begin. Everything else follows from that.

In the Tai Chi tradition, there is a concept called beginners mind, the understanding that the most experienced practitioners approach their practice with the same openness and curiosity as someone doing it for the very first time. Not because they have not learned anything, but because they understand that the practice is always deeper than wherever they currently are within it. There is always more to discover in the next breath, in the next movement, in the next quiet ten minutes.

You are not finished. You are beginning.

The chair is ready. The breath is available. The practice is waiting, exactly where you left it.

Come back to it tomorrow.

With gratitude for the courage it takes to care for yourself,

Your Chair Tai Chi Instructor

Acknowledgements

A book about the practice of moving together could not have been written alone.

My deepest gratitude goes to the hundreds of students I have had the privilege of teaching across fifteen years in community centers, rehabilitation facilities, and retirement homes. You taught me infinitely more than I taught you. Your resilience, your humor, your willingness to try something new in the most challenging seasons of your lives shaped every word of this program. This book exists because of what you showed me was possible.

To the physical therapists, occupational therapists, geriatric physicians, and healthcare professionals who generously shared their clinical expertise and trusted this practice enough to recommend it to their patients; your collaboration made this program safer, deeper, and more effective than it could ever have been without you.

To the global Tai Chi community whose devotion has preserved this art across generations, this book stands on your shoulders with respect.

To my colleagues in senior wellness who offered encouragement throughout this process, your support is reflected on every page.

To my own teachers who first placed these movements in my hands, I carry your instruction with me always.

Thank you. All of you.

— Xian Ming

About the Author

Xian Ming is a Certified Tai Chi and Qi Gong Instructor with a lifelong dedication to one purpose: helping older adults move better, live more freely, and age with confidence and dignity.

Over fifteen years of practice have taken Xian into community centers, retirement communities, and rehabilitation facilities, working directly with seniors navigating arthritis, chronic pain, balance challenges, anxiety, and mild cognitive decline. That depth of real-world experience shapes every page of this book.

Xian works in close collaboration with physical therapists, occupational therapists, and geriatric healthcare professionals to ensure every movement program meets the highest standards of safety and clinical relevance for older adults. This interdisciplinary approach has made Xian's chair-based Tai Chi and Qi Gong programs among the most trusted in senior wellness settings.

But beyond the credentials, what defines Xian's teaching is something simpler: a genuine belief that everybody, at every age, deserves a practice that meets it with patience, respect, and care.

Bonus: The 10-Minute Daily Quick Reference Guide

Feel free to photocopy or print these pages, snap a picture of them with your smartphone, or simply lay the book flat near your chair. This way, you can move continuously through your daily 10-minute sessions without ever needing to break your concentration to flip pages.

How to Use These Guide (Quick Start Rule)

To get the best results; better balance, less stiffness, and a clearer mind, consistency is quite important. Here is your simple roadmap:

- **Frequency: 5 days a week.** You do not need to practice every day.

- **Rest Days: 2 days off.** Take these whenever your body needs a break (for example, take weekends off, or rest every third day). Listen to your joints.

- **Duration: 10 minutes a day.** Do not rush. If you move slowly and it takes 12 minutes, that is perfect.

- **Best Time to Practice: Mid-Morning (9:00 AM – 11:00 AM).** This allows your body to shake off morning stiffness before you get tired. *(If you prefer evenings, practice 1 hour before bed to wind down).*

- **Repetitions:** The numbers listed below (e.g., "4 to 6 cycles, circles, etc.") are just suggestions. If 3 feels like enough for the movement, then stop at 3. Never push through pain.

Week 1: Gentle Introduction to Movements

Preparation (1 Minute)

- Sit forward on your chair, feet flat on the floor, hip-width apart.

- Find your posture: spine tall, shoulders dropped, hands resting in your lap.

- Take 3 slow, deep belly breaths (inhale through the nose, exhale through the mouth).

1. The Warm-Up (3 Minutes)

Movement	Action	Visual Reference
Neck Rolls	2 slow half-circles in each direction (forward arc only).	*Chin to chest* 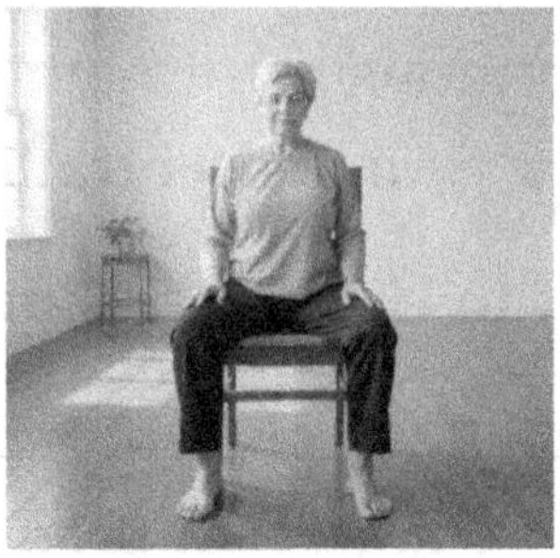 *Right ear to right shoulder* 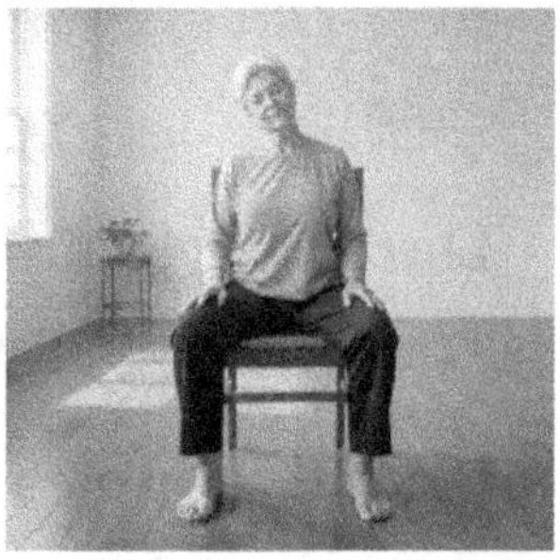 *Left ear to left shoulder* 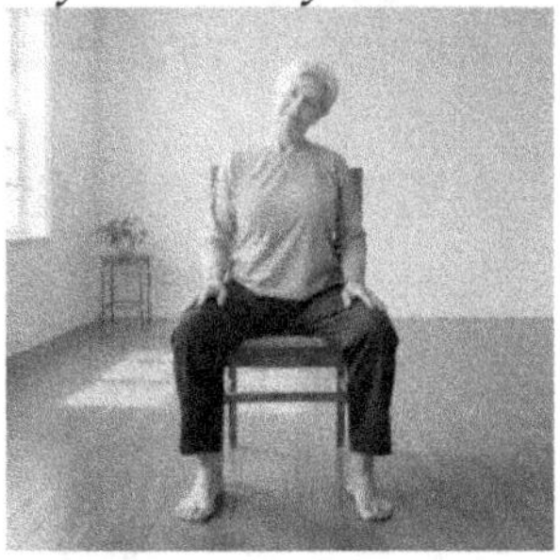
Shoulder Rolls	3 to 4 slow circles backward, then 3 to 4 slow circles forward.	*Shoulders up* 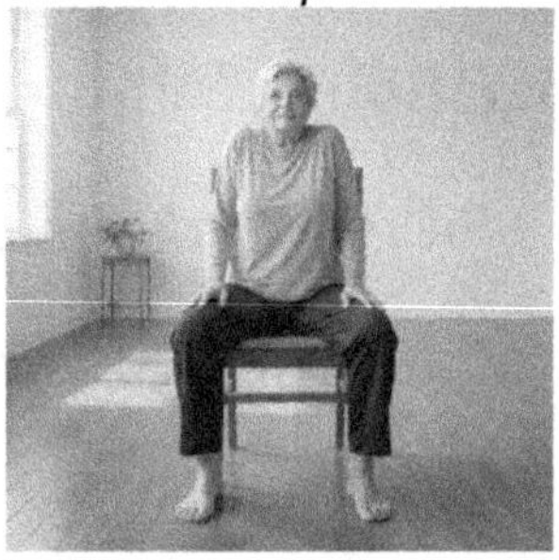

Movement	Action	Visual Reference
		Shoulders rolling back/down 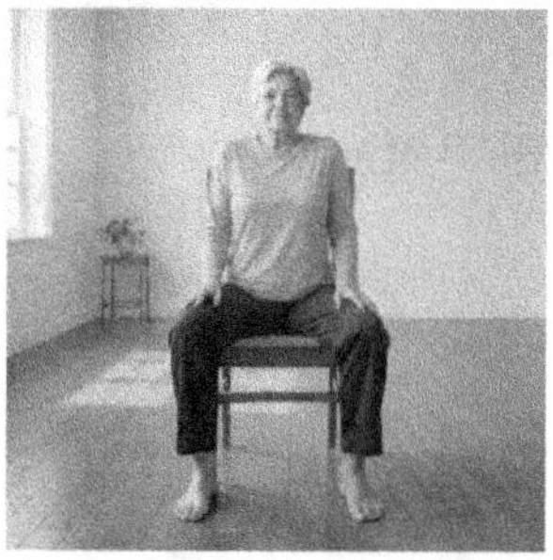
Wrist Flexions & Circles	5 to 6 flexions (down and up), then 5 circles in each direction.	*Wrists flexed down* 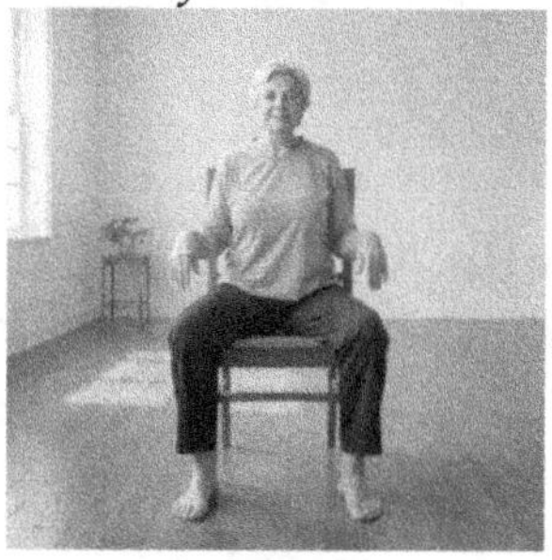 *Wrists flexed up* 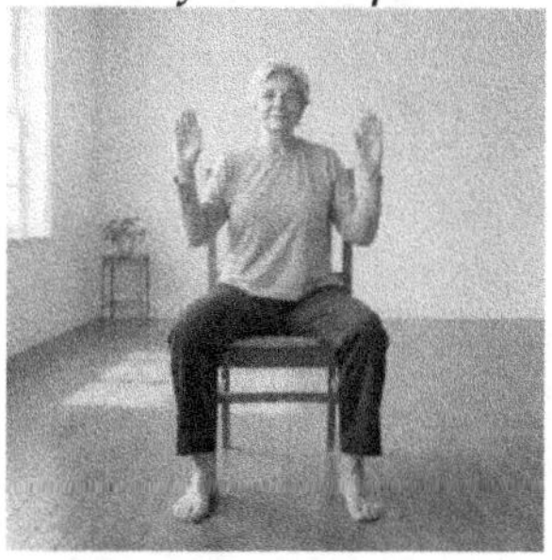 *Wrist circles* 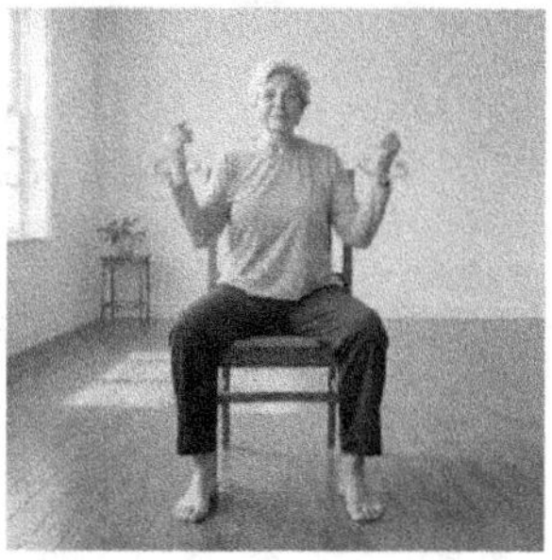

2. The Core Movements (5 Minutes)

Movement	Action	Visual Reference
Basic Breathing	Place one hand on chest, one on belly. 5 to 6 deep breath cycles, letting the belly rise and fall.	*(No image needed, focus hands on chest and belly)*
Gentle Arm Swings	4 to 6 full cycles. **Inhale:** arms float up. **Exhale:** arms float down.	*Inhale - Arms floating forward/up* *Exhale - Arms floating down*
Seated Forward Bends	3 to 4 slow, gentle bends. Take a full inhale before bending forward. **Exhale:** fold forward. **Inhale:** rise back up.	*Exhale - Fold forward* *Inhale - Rise up*

Movement	Action	Visual Reference

The Closing (1 Minute)

- Rest your hands in your lap. Sit quietly for 30 to 60 seconds.

- Notice how your body feels. Take one final deep breath before standing up slowly.

Week 2: Increasing Mobility and Flexibility

Preparation & Warm-Up (2 Minutes)

- **Preparation:** Sit tall, feet flat, spine lengthened. Take 3 slow, deep belly breaths.

- **Warm-Up:** Perform Week 1 quick Neck Rolls, Shoulder Rolls, and Wrist Circles to loosen the joints.

The Core Movements (7 Minutes)

Movement	Action	Visual Reference
Seated Gentle Twists	3 to 4 twists per side (left and right side). Take a full inhale without beginning the rotation. **Exhale:** turn left gently. **Inhale:** return to center.	*Exhale - Turning left*

Movement	Action	Visual Reference
	Exhale: turn right gently. **Inhale:** return to center.	*Inhale - Returned to center*
Breath & Reach	4 to 6 alternating cycles. **Inhale:** arms reach up and over. **Exhale:** arms drawn down.	*Inhale - Arms reaching up and over* *Exhale - Arms draw inward across chest*
Seated Leg Raises	3 to 5 cycles, alternating sides (right and left side). **Inhale:** extend leg. **Exhale:** lower foot.	*Inhale - Right leg extended*

Movement	Action	Visual Reference
		Exhale - Right leg lowered 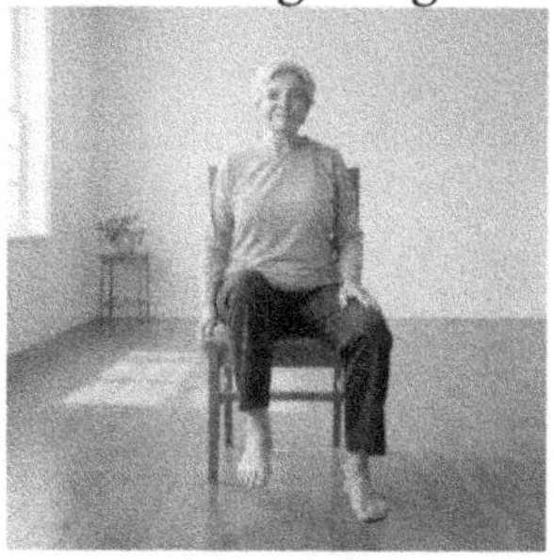
Seated Hip Circles	3 to 4 slow rotations in each direction on each side (right and left side).	*Right knee raised in a small, slow circle* 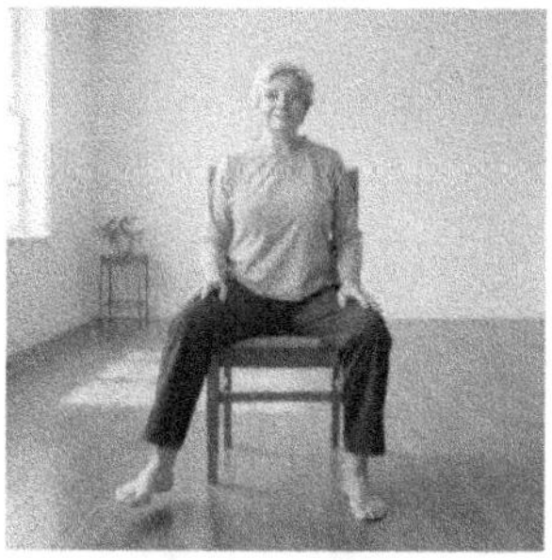 *Right knee circling* 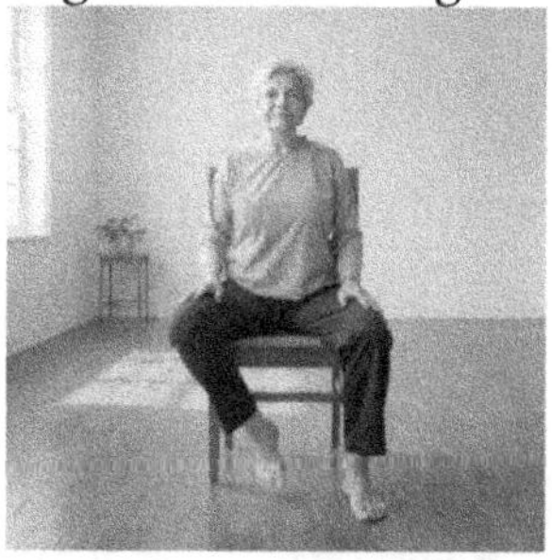
Slow Side-to-Side	4 to 6 full side-to-side cycles. **Inhale:** shift right. **Exhale:** return to center. **Inhale:** shift left.	*Inhale - Shifting right* 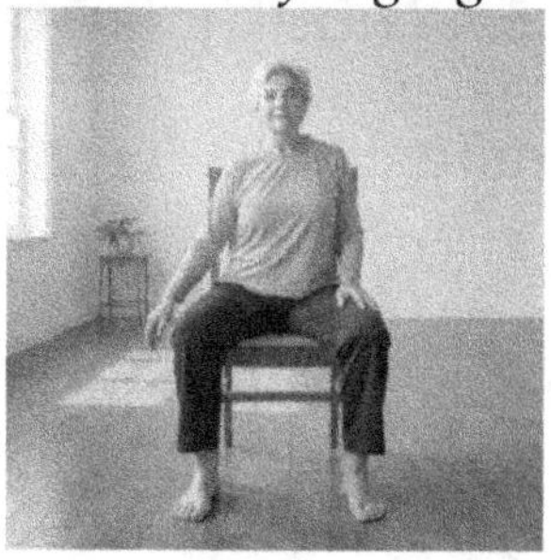 *Exhale - Return center*

Movement	Action	Visual Reference
		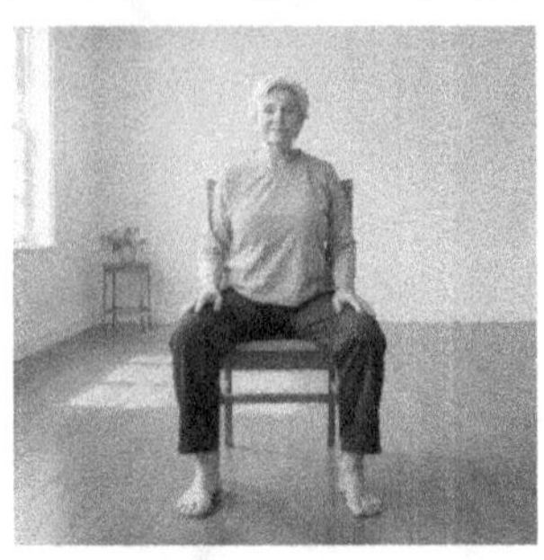

Inhale - Shifting left

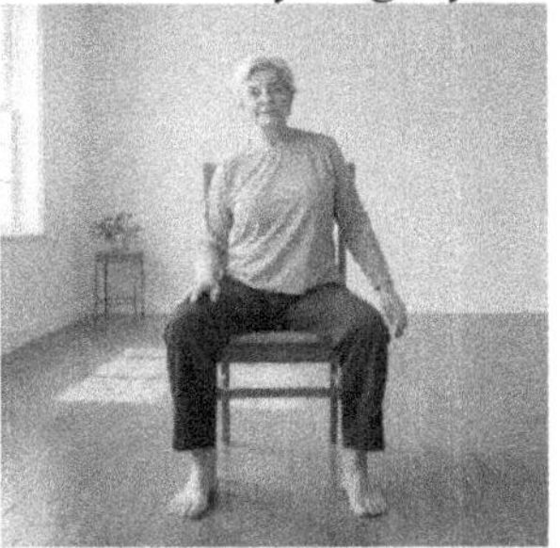

The Closing (1 Minute)

- Return to neutral posture. Hands resting in your lap.

- Close your eyes softly for 30 to 60 seconds. Notice the new circulation in your legs and spine. Breathe naturally before rising.

Week 3: Strengthening and Coordination

Preparation & Warm-Up (2 Minutes)

- **Preparation:** Sit tall, feet flat, spine lengthened. Take 3 slow, deep belly breaths.

- **Warm-Up:** Perform your standard Week 1 Warm-Up (Neck, Shoulders, Wrists).

The Core Movements (7 Minutes)

Movement	Action	Visual Reference
Seated Cloud Hands	6 to 8 full continuous cycles (3 to 4 twists per side – right and left side). Let the waist turn the arms.	*Inhale - Right hand high/ Right side twist* 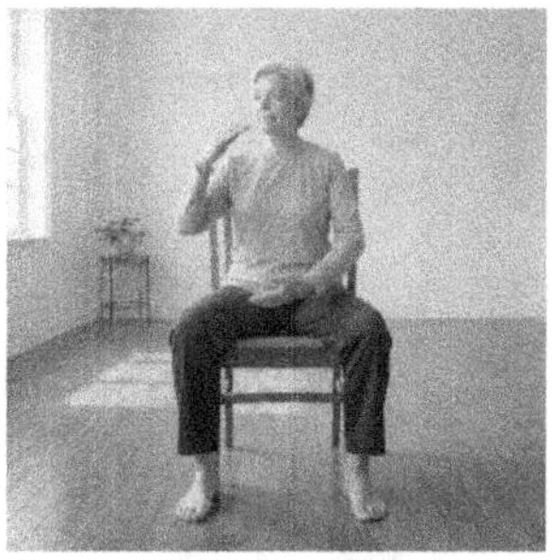 *Exhale - Left hand high/ Left side twist* 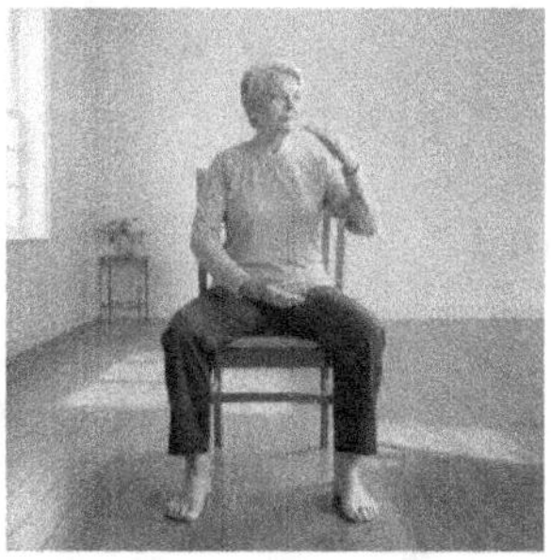
Knee Lifts & Strokes	4 to 6 alternating cycles. **Inhale:** raise right knee and left arm forward. **Exhale:** raise left knee and right arm forward.	*Inhale - Right knee up, , left arm forward* 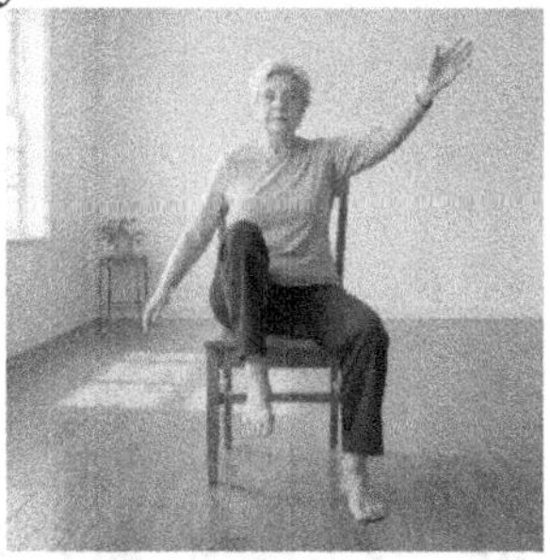 *Exhale - Left knee up, right arm forward*

Movement	Action	Visual Reference
		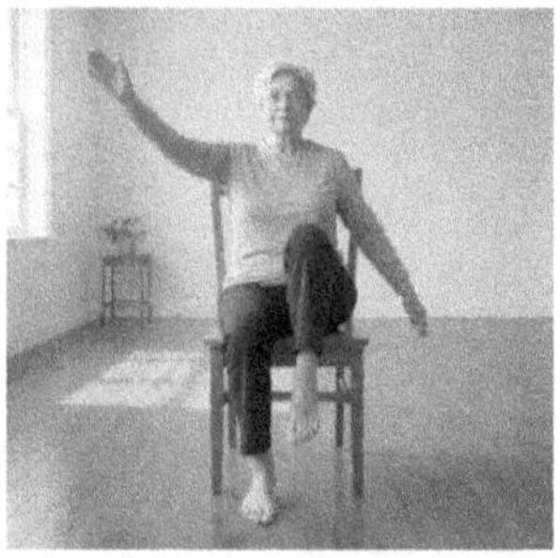 *Inhale - Raising right arm/knee*
Golden Rooster Stand	3 to 4 holds per side. Pause and repeat on the other side. **Inhale:** raise right arm and right knee. **Exhale:** lower right arm and knee.	*Inhale - Raising left arm/knee*
		Inhale - Right hand behind right ear
Chair Tai Chi Brush Knee	3 to 4 cycles per side. **Inhale:** raise one hand behind the ear, opposite hand rests on thigh. **Exhale:** brush one hand over knee while pushing other hand forward.	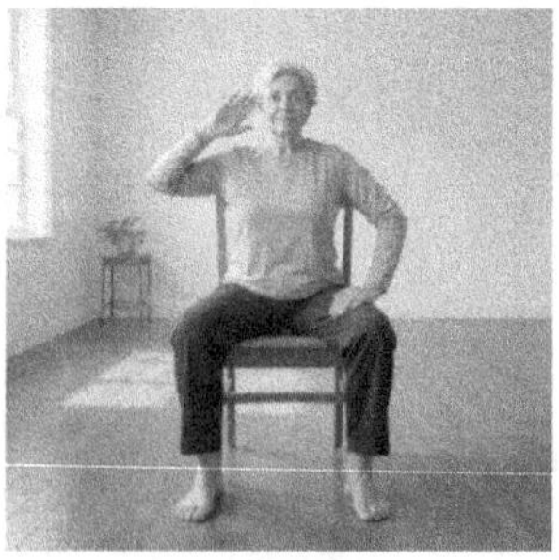 *Left hand brushing right knee*

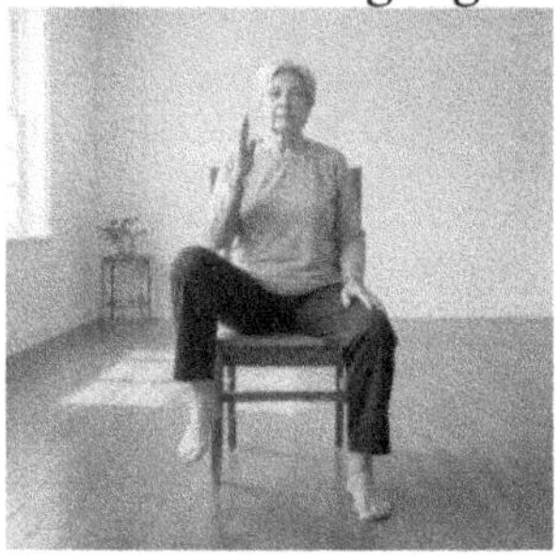

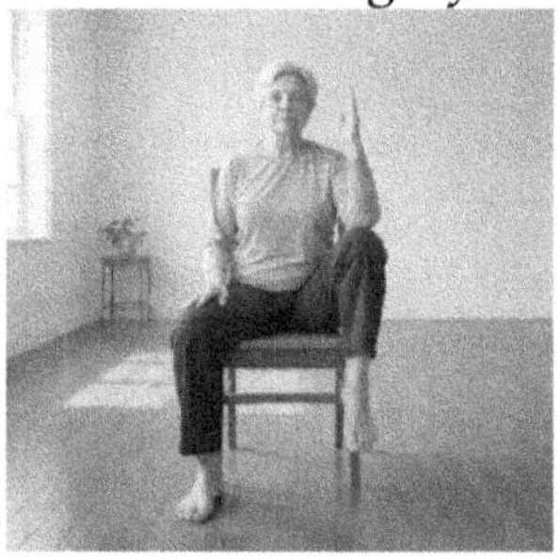

Movement	Action	Visual Reference

Exhale - Right hand forward / Left hand fully brushed over right knee

The Closing (1 Minute)

- Rest your hands heavily on your thighs.

- Sit in stillness for 30 to 60 seconds. Observe the coordination and warmth generated in your body. Take one deep clearing breath.

Week 4: Fluidity and Mental Focus

Preparation & Warm-Up (2 Minutes)

- **Preparation:** Sit tall, feet flat, spine lengthened.

- **Warm-Up:** Perform Week 1 standard warm-up (Neck, Shoulder, and Wrist rolls).

The Core Flow (7 Minutes)

Movement	Action	Visual Reference
Leg Extensions with Flow	8 to 10 continuous, alternating cycles. **Inhale:** right leg extends and slowly returns. **Exhale:** left leg begins extension—*no pausing.*	*Inhale - Right leg extends and slowly returns* 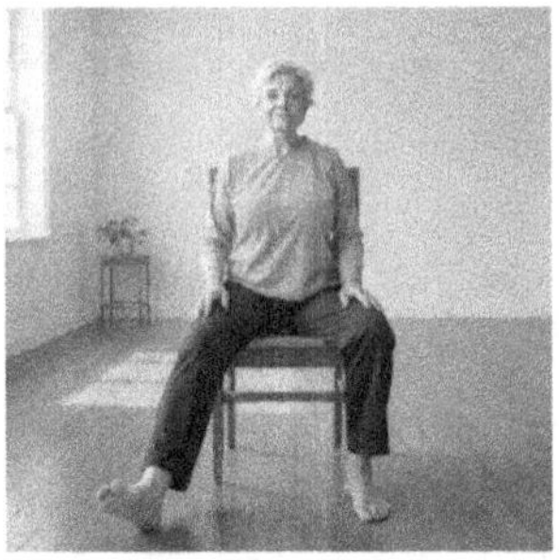 *Exhale - Left leg begins extension—no pausing* 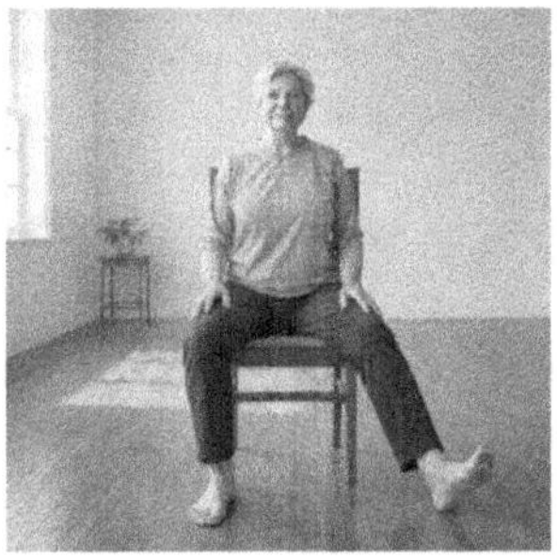
Tai Chi Push Movements	4 to 6 full 3-directional cycles. **Inhale:** hands at rest. **Exhale:** push hand forward. **Inhale:** twist and lift wrists upward. **Exhale:** twist and press downward.	*Inhale - Hands at rest* 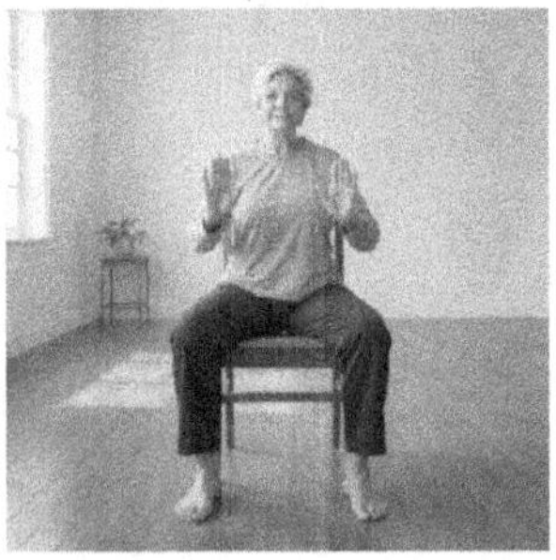

Movement	Action	Visual Reference
		Push forward 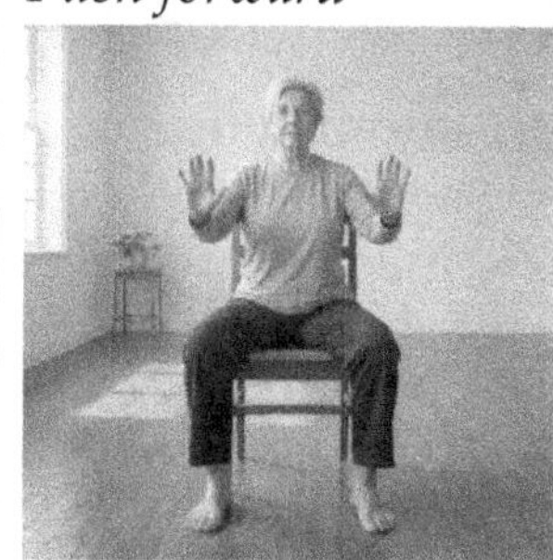 *Inhale – Twist and lift wrists upward* 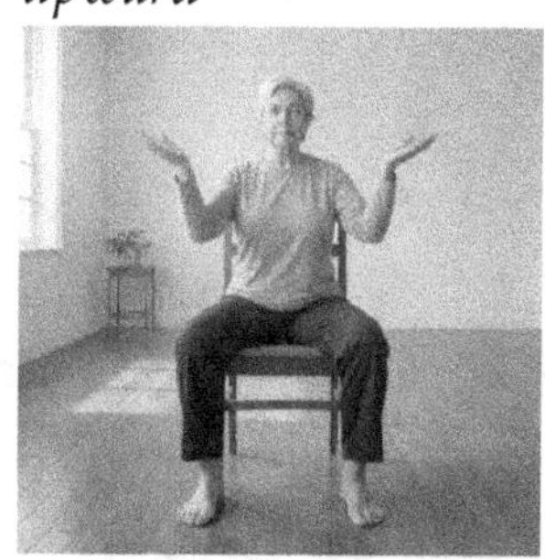 *Exhale - Twist and press wrists downward* 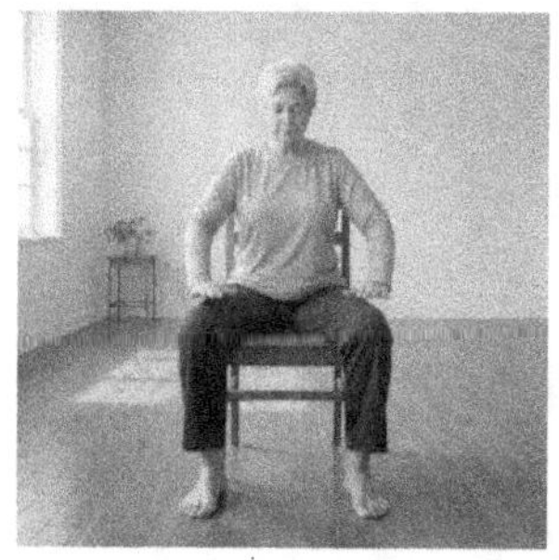
Seated Cloud Hands + "Warm River"	Perform 6 to 8 continuous cycles while imagining your hands moving slowly through a warm river. Let the gentle resistance naturally slow your movement.	*(Use Week 3 Cloud Hands images as mental reference)*

The Closing (1 Minute)

- Return to a perfectly still, seated posture.

- Reflect on your chosen Visualization for 30 to 60 seconds. Notice the stillness in your mind and the ease in your joints.

- Acknowledge the time you gave to yourself today. Stand up slowly and deliberately.